on the

Burning Out
on the COVID Front Lines

A Doctor's Memoir of Fatherhood,
Race and Perseverance
in the Pandemic

Dhaval R. Desai, M.D.

McFarland & Company, Inc., Publishers
Jefferson, North Carolina

ISBN (print) 978-1-4766-9182-4
ISBN (ebook) 978-1-4766-5111-8

LIBRARY OF CONGRESS AND BRITISH LIBRARY
CATALOGUING DATA ARE AVAILABLE

Library of Congress Control Number 2023024517

Printed in the United States of America

*McFarland & Company, Inc., Publishers
Box 611, Jefferson, North Carolina 28640
www.mcfarlandpub.com*

To Yogita, Kaiya, and Kaveh,
who have been my rock and sun
through the pandemic and beyond.
I love you.

I also dedicate this book to all the frontline healthcare workers
who have sacrificed so much personally and professionally
during the pandemic and beyond.
And to my healthcare colleagues across the world
who are no longer with us,
you will be remembered and celebrated as heroes forever.

Contents

Prologue

Late spring, 2021. A steady trickle of patients with routine complaints of chest pain, falls and fevers had been arriving in the ER triage area throughout the afternoon when a red sedan rapidly pulled in. A man who looked to be in his eighties was in the passenger seat, visibly coughing. The driver, middle-aged and without a mask, scurried out and flagged a triage nurse for help.

"My dad is having trouble breathing and having fevers. He can't get out of the car. Get me a wheelchair now!" The nurse brought around a wheelchair and started helping the elderly patient into it.

"Sir, I'm going to help you get into the emergency room, and here's a mask I need you to put on before we go in."

His groggy eyes opened wide. Becoming angry, he screamed, "Whatever! I don't want a mask!" The nurse pleaded with him until at last he agreed, but he wore it loose, below his nose.

While the nurse registered the patient, the son walked in with his sister and elderly mother, all without masks. When asked to put them on, the son shot back, "Oh, here we go again! These freaking masks don't work, and y'all have this ridiculous policy!" Security then presented the rules to him as an ultimatum. His mother, it turns out, was also feeling weak: she had a constant cough and had bouts of vomiting earlier in the day.

The triage nurse checked them in and proceeded to escort them to the room when they mentioned they had been to a family gathering a week ago and two of their family members had coronavirus. Both mother and father then were placed in separate rooms and put on contact isolation. The husband needed oxygen immediately. The wife needed IV fluids, as her blood pressure was low. When the son and daughter were told they could not remain with their parents due to possible coronavirus and the need to isolate, the hospital staff was broadsided with "This is such crap! My parents don't have coronavirus. It's a hoax. The vaccines, the masks ... all of it!"

The family angrily departed while the ER team quickly triaged and worked up the two new patients. They were sick and needed to be admitted. A rapid COVID PCR test was positive for each, and my team was called to admit them to the hospital for further care. Reviewing their history, labs, and the fact that they were both in their eighties, I worried, perplexed, about how sick they were and what this meant for their prognoses.

I walked into the elderly male's full isolation room wearing a yellow isolation gown, tight N95 mask, eye goggles and face shield. When I tried to explain what my role was, he vehemently cut in, "I can't understand you through that mask. Take it off!" I refused and assured him I would protect myself. Giving me one- and two-word answers— he was short of breath and coughing—he balked when asked if he had obtained the vaccine for the coronavirus this year.

"No! We don't believe in it." His response was a dismissal. He closed his eyes and turned away from me.

His wife, for her part, was so weak that she wouldn't even fully awaken to talk with me.

I called the son of these two patients for more information and perhaps some insight. Hopeful for partnership and support to help care for his parents, I was met with the opposite.

"No, Doctor, none of us are vaccinated, and we don't believe in it. Do not give them any of those experimental drugs like remdesivir! Just keep it simple. This isn't a big deal. They're going to be fine. We know it!"

I could feel my blood boil with anger and frustration but held back. I wanted to tell him how insulting his views were—not just to me but to all of my colleagues who have been on the front line for the past sixteen months. Instead, all I could say was, "We will do the best we can," and hung up.

Prologue

More than a year into the pandemic and even now, yet again, I am faced with two unvaccinated elderly patients and a family who believed neither in the virus, its vaccine, nor any life-saving treatment for it.

CHAPTER ONE

A New Virus

February 23, 2020, 7:36 a.m.

Our newborn son was fast asleep in the bassinet next to the hospital bed. Yogita and I had just fallen asleep. We'd been up all night, coordinating feeding, changing diapers, going through different hospital assessments. The new morning nurse poked her head in to say hi and put her name on the dry-erase board. Barely awake and groggy, Yogita smiled and whispered hello. My eyes were dry from sleeping with my contacts in, and my throat felt scratchy from the hospital air. I could see the outline of my wife's head leaning against the headrail with the small light near the sink. She was sleepy but still had that glow as she looked down at our baby boy. Even though we'd been through this before with our daughter, on this quiet morning it all felt brand new.

Though nauseous from a combination of exhaustion, stress and adrenaline, underneath we felt the soft feelings of new parenthood: wonder, tenderness, gratefulness, joy. With the arrival of Kaveh, our new son, at last our family of four felt complete. A promising year lay ahead, and with it, a sense of hope, enlightenment and excitement.

I had just enough time to grab a coffee from the hospital lobby before I was due back to my wife and son. That morning we were to meet with the lactation consultant and prepare for discharge the following day. In the background, *Good Morning America* was on the small TV mounted on the wall, the chyron breaking news about a novel coronavirus.

Kaveh was in my arms, wrapped in a few swaddle blankets too many, opening and closing his dark brown eyes while my wife ate bland oatmeal. The TV screen kept cutting to images of the *Diamond*

Princess, a cruise ship now quarantined with coronavirus cases, and more new cases were beginning to appear in Seattle and Oregon. I'd heard about the situation in Wuhan and Italy, and even now, seeing it in the western corner of the United States, it just seemed far away. It wouldn't make its way to Georgia. This would be quickly contained.

Coronaviruses, I knew, are here already. I'd seen different forms of the virus in pediatric populations during my training. It manifests with routine symptoms and is categorized as the common cold. I continued watching *Good Morning America*, assuming that this new coronavirus would be no different. As a doctor and director of hospital medicine and a leader to other physicians, I felt I would know if this were truly worrisome.

A story, after all, is always *breaking news*; how better to capture our attention and keep us riveted? This breaking news reminded me of a promise I'd made, that these next ten days were going to be different. My family had just grown, and I was determined to not be consumed by competing problems and situations at the hospital. I had supremely talented and capable colleagues covering me. This was my time with family. As the news went to commercials, my thoughts went to my son. *I love you.* I gazed down at him. *I will always protect you.*

That morning, I experienced the routine of hospital dynamics and flow but from the other side: nurses, a visit from the pediatrician and OB-GYN, paperwork. The number of hospital workers who entered our room—upwards of twenty, each with a different job to do, all within twenty-four hours—was uncanny. We all interacted happily with one another, with smiles and handshakes, as in any other normal day.

Our room was almost always full. Kaiya, our four-year-old daughter, had visited the previous day with both sets of grandparents. When I took her in to meet her new brother, her eyes grew wide and she gripped my hand tighter. With a big smile and a squeal, she started jumping up and down then hurried to the bassinet and gently whispered, "Hi, baby. I'm your big sister." My wife and I locked eyes as the new big sister gently patted her new brother. When it was time for a feeding, Kaiya—who had been holding the baby under close supervision—refused to give him up, thinking she could do it as she did with her dolls at home. Worried about her adjustment, we made sure to give Kaiya extra love in those first early days.

I noticed that at one point, we had six adults, a four-year-old child and a brand-new baby crammed into one small room. Remodeled yet still tiny, the room was designed for a new mother and her baby, with one side couch for a family member. On ours, the grandparents were all jammed together, passing the baby from one to the other. I was nervous about germs and exposures. (A newborn's immune system has yet to develop.) While the baby was being held by one of the grandmothers, my father let out a dry cough. Taking no chances, I requested that he wash his hands immediately and sanitize with alcohol. That we were packed together in a hospital room, breathing on one another while admiring this new baby, was nerve-racking. From my work in pediatrics, I had seen a fair share of newborns sick in the first weeks of life and I worried that my son would be one of them.

* * *

Discharged and now back home.

As we organized ourselves, unpacking from the hospital, we had the news on in the background. Again, I heard about the novel coronavirus. This time, though, I felt a degree of concern from a world public health standpoint, with cases and deaths increasing around the globe, yet we've always been so privileged and protected here in the States, and I predicted that would hold. Regardless, my focus now was on my family. They deserved my attention, and I was trying hard to avoid any thoughts related to work. The hospital—and the novel coronavirus—could wait.

At home, I was overwhelmed. I had to learn to navigate and divide my attention; Kaiya, for her part, wasn't used to sharing the spotlight. That was a challenge. Chaos had become the new normal. Sleepless nights continued as my son adjusted to life outside the womb, and our daughter would still come running into our room in the middle of the night. Mornings were taken up by first fixing breakfast, getting Kaiya ready and dropping her off at preschool, then helping with the baby's changing, burping and holding. In a blink, afternoon would arrive before I'd even had coffee. Laundry seemed endless, especially since we washed the baby's things separately with hypoallergenic detergent. Preparing meals without interruption was impossible. All day long I'd be putting out fires, and any kind of planning had to take this into account.

Days blurred together in a sleep-deprived state, every powernap short-lived. Yogita had the harder role with nursing (and all other maternal demands), clearly adjusting more adeptly than I. Through it all, we were blessed to have my parents nearby, as well as my mother-in-law staying for two weeks—which meant, of course, that we didn't learn how to function alone with two children for the first few weeks. I remembered how friends would say, "the first few weeks of newborn life lead to amnesia: when you do it again, it's as if you have no recollection of what it was like." No truer words.

Yet, despite my attempts to solely focus on things at home, I could feel the outside pressure mounting, that things were subtly starting to change. More and more, my thoughts were of the hospital. My mind would drift when burping Kaveh or loading the dishwasher, and inevitably I would scroll, scanning headlines on my phone, wondering as the buzz became louder about this virus. I did resist the urge to check work email and did not click on the blue envelope for updates. That was a major challenge. *Everyone's* focus, it seemed, was shifting.

As one week of paternity leave finished, coronavirus coverage nationwide increased. What the virus could do and where it was spreading was a subject of much speculation. Around the second of March I began to worry. My team is on the front line. What would we do if someone had it at our hospital? I started receiving texts from colleagues asking how prepared we were for patients coming in with possible coronavirus. They posed questions to which I had no answers. I said we had to align with the broader health system and follow all guidance. I reassured team members I would be back the following week and promised to communicate developments in the meantime. Alarm bells were starting to ring. This was turning into a potentially serious event.

For better or worse, our family usually has the TV running in the background when we're at home. Evenings typically are cartoons that my daughter loves, but during the day, it's news all the time. My wife, although on maternity leave, continued to check her emails and wanted to keep tabs on her work as a physician in physical medicine and rehabilitation. To see her spend hours on patient-related issues outside of work is not at all unusual; she has a passion to give the best patient care and maintain the most professional relationships with her patients and colleagues. We both worked within the same health system and always chatted about the latest happenings.

Knowing my style, she then asked me, "Are you looking at these emails about the coronavirus? Should you be doing something?"

I held her hand, smoothed her hair, and said something about needing to draw boundaries with work during this important time at home right now. She smiled in that way that says *okay* but raised her eyebrows and semi-smirked, knowing that I was fighting the urge to get to work.

While my mind and energies were focused on my family, admittedly I was starting to obsess. What if there were COVID cases in the metro Atlanta area? What if a patient who was traveling abroad showed up at our ER with COVID-like symptoms? Still, I felt part of a system that was prepared. A few years earlier, two cases of Ebola were treated at one of our hospitals. If we could deal with that, we could deal with a coronavirus. We had prepared with a whole triage plan that time, and when I was in residency, I was part of the H1N1 flu outbreak. I had seen these viruses that caused hype and hysteria, and each time, I was always secure and protected.

Why would this time be any different?

CHAPTER TWO

Surge

My ten days of paternity leave quickly ended. Yogita would remain at home with our son, while my daughter would continue at preschool. My in-laws were heading back to Maryland, and I was looking forward to our new routine.

Leading up to my return to work, I prioritized items to work on. Determining the status of the coronavirus—what we were seeing in the city and country—was high on the list. During that time, I was briefed on a plan to transfer potential patients with symptoms to the bigger university-based hospital, where they would be treated in a specialized contained area. This sounded reasonable and still felt like a back-up plan we wouldn't need to utilize. Excited to be getting back, I looked forward to helping however I could. To me, the hospital felt like a second home. It's where I belonged.

* * *

I didn't need an alarm that morning, March 9. I was awake at six and got my daughter ready for preschool so Yogita could get a few more minutes of sleep between cluster feedings. Despite my sleep deprivation, I was energized, excited to be going back to work. The drive to the hospital felt normal, nothing new. After settling in, I headed to one of the acute care floors, phone in hand, to catch up with everyone and share pictures I had picked out of Kaveh.

Several members of the care team were huddled in a way that made them seem more like football players than healthcare workers. I asked a doctor friend what was going on. Yellow tape and isolation gowns were plastered to the door to a room, with a sign that read "SEE NURSE BEFORE ENTERING." A box of gloves was wedged beside the door.

"That patient is positive."

*   *   *

Soon after came a steady stream of patients—of all ages—presenting with complaints suggestive of the novel coronavirus: weakness, fevers, severe cough and gasps from shortness of breath. The first weeks of March were filled with meetings, all with dynamic new pieces of information garnered from other sources. My phone dinged incessantly with calendar invitations for yet another meeting or huddle, more and more of which were being scheduled online or conducted via cell phone. Mornings were filled caring for patients, with meetings about departmental issues such as personal protective equipment (PPE) conservation and navigating clinical guideline updates. A daily afternoon huddle would bring all issues and updates together as the day wrapped up, only to filter down again to my team. It was chaos, the situation changing by the hour, but, in the midst of it, the only way I knew to remotely stay organized was to communicate frequently and candidly with my group. I was persistent in the messaging that things would only become more dynamic.

My coworkers showed up with their game face on, ready to take on the next challenge in this burgeoning health crisis. I developed a newfound respect for every hospital multidisciplinary leader with whom I worked: not only doctors and nurses but respiratory therapists, dieticians, physical therapists, infection prevention specialists and all who were there pitching in. Despite their overwhelming stress and fatigue, their determination and energy to carry their respective staff through the unfolding pandemic was palpable: each was vested and well-intended in doing what was right for patients and staff, and to witness this collaboration was magical. There were no antagonisms; whatever one team lacked or wherever they fell short, another would quickly step in and provide.

Even so, our reality was that information varied by the hour as to treatment guidelines, PPE availability and isolation protocols, all of which required constant adjustment and modifications. Due to shortages of isolation gowns, the hospital had to adapt to reusing plastic surgical gowns by sanitizing them. Masking at first was not mandatory, and even when required, N95 masks were only used initially for confirmed COVID-19 cases and not for those still awaiting test results. In my case, since I have a short beard, I had to adapt to wearing a Controlled Air Purifying Respirator (CAPR) device that was shared among many. (The CAPR is worn with constant air circulation and resembles the headgear of an astronaut suit.) Often, I felt I was competing with other staff for access to protective equipment, as there were only six CAPR devices in the hospital, and they tend to break down and frequently need charging. Some days, I would share the same device with a colleague, trading off every few hours.

Before the pandemic, one personal strength I could always rely on was my ability to communicate with my group. Leading a team of hospital physicians focused on the care of acutely ill patients had always been rewarding. We work together on the front line, over the long haul. Not only does it make me feel grounded, but working closely alongside my team also helps to build relationships with staff and patients. Not having all the answers, I find it satisfying and gratifying to help navigate physicians toward the best outcome, whatever the scenario and challenge, and now, with COVID-19, I needed to be especially transparent. Never before had I communicated so much by email or responded to so many texts and phone calls. Sometimes this consisted of merely listening to the frustration, fear and angst felt by most of us with the daily unknowns—conversations that were just as therapeutic for me, as I too shared similar anxieties and fears about what might come next. What earlier would have been a monthly staff meeting with a few general updates outside of an unexpected crisis was now replaced with daily emails updating my team on the latest. As some of the information appeared redundant, I wondered if I was overcommunicating and exhausting everyone, but silence can be deafening—especially in a crisis—and I refused to be quiet during this time. My team expected to hear from me.

The clinical stigmata of patients with COVID-19 were quite distinct. I spent years in training learning disease processes, patterns and treatment, and I felt comfortable and confident treating acutely ill patients in the hospital. It had become my bread and butter. But this pandemic was different. Patients presenting with mild respiratory symptoms were showing unique lung changes on chest X-rays. They would report having a cough and shortness of breath and of not being able to catch their breath. Specifically, many described a drowning sensation as they started to feel worse, accompanied by a kind of "air hunger" where they felt they could not get enough oxygen into their lungs. None of this was alleviated by rest. In addition, countless patients could not taste or smell. Intractable back pain and headaches plagued many who never experienced such issues before.

The majority of COVID patients who arrived at the hospital came on the sixth or seventh day of feeling ill. This indicated a time frame where symptoms were peaking and felt to be at their worst, a pattern not typically seen with other common pneumonias and respiratory infections. Even those patients with milder disease exhibited such despair with their suffering associated with shortness of breath, weakness and muscle aches. Their chest X-rays showed distinct infiltrates at the bases that were seen over and over in patients of all ages. A thirty-five-year-old with no major medical issues should not typically get a pneumonia that causes such lung damage, yet this was repeatedly the pattern.

I was used to treating a geriatric patient population, but patients with COVID-19 represented all adult age groups. It was a harsh wake-up call that this disease could affect any one of us when I started seeing thirty- and forty-year-old patients admitted with COVID-19. Some cases were milder, patients who required lower amounts of oxygen but were plagued with weakness and body aches, along with an inability to keep themselves hydrated, which led to longer hospitalizations. Other patients were so severely short of breath that they could not talk without gasping, unable even to adjust themselves in bed without their oxygen levels dropping to the 70s or 80s (we typically want it above 90). Going from room to room, I would see a cohort of patients with COVID-19 whose symptoms were different but whose eyes locked onto mine with the same degree of fear and suffering.

About two weeks after finishing paternity leave, I was changing my son's diaper early one Saturday morning when I received a call from a colleague who sounded frantic. They had to intervene when a patient (now on her fourth day of hospitalization) who had been stable on a small amount of oxygen and expected to be discharged soon cried out in misery that she "couldn't catch her breath" and felt as though she was "drowning." The patient was rushed to the ICU and quickly placed on a ventilator. A few hours later, her test came back positive, four days into her hospitalized state as a patient under investigation for COVID-19. In the first weeks of the pandemic, it was so confusing, as we really did not know who was positive or negative for COVID-19; testing took days. Were we to assume everyone was positive? If yes, we certainly did not have enough PPE to treat accordingly. As I decompressed with my colleague, it was clear that this turn was unexpected.

All I could think about that Saturday morning was, how many more patients would end up like this? What was it about this virus that was so different—and what else might we not be able to predict? Also, were healthcare workers being exposed to this virus more frequently than initially thought?

Not only was the disease process of COVID-19 unpredictable, but we also found we were stuck on how to treat it. Clinical practice guidelines were changing and evolving. I was glued to my phone for updates and took part in several professional groups on social media where we discussed similar patient scenarios. Hydroxychloroquine had mixed reviews, and we were not convinced it was the miracle drug. Elected officials at the time were claiming victory with hydroxychloroquine, and a great many patients bought into that. Steroids initially were not recommended, then later changed to strongly recommended. Remdesivir was emerging as a popular option but we were advised to follow strict criteria for its utilization.

Hospitalized patients began demanding hydroxychloroquine and remdesivir for treatment as though they were choosing from a fast-food menu. I had never before observed so many patients demand such specific drugs and treatments; it stemmed from desperation, and I found it exhausting to have the same conversation over and over about appropriate use. I stood my ground, insisting to certain patients that

I would not prescribe them hydroxychloroquine. Some would respect my decision while others would counter it and threaten to leave. (None did—it was clear their fear of getting worse from COVID was greater than their pride and strength of their convictions.) I had to stay aligned with our treatment guidelines. There is certainly more than one way to treat most disease processes, but now was not the time to begin varying practices. There was a degree of mistrust and skepticism about COVID-19 and the pandemic, and any variation or inconsistency in practice would only create more of it. The right thing to do was to continue to be unified as a group.

While we struggled to treat, the question remained how best to protect ourselves from COVID-19. As to PPE—and there was never enough—we were in complete conservation mode. This was a firm message sent by leadership across the system and felt across the country. Gone were the days where I used one N95 mask per patient per day; we now used them until they were completely unusable from moisture, worn straps, or visible stains. Sometimes the mask was changed daily, other times, every few days. A nurse in charge of conserving PPE once questioned why I needed a fresh mask when I got a new one the day before. She didn't know that in the interim I had visited eighteen different COVID rooms, sometimes twice. While all I wanted to do was yell at her for even questioning me, I simply told her it was worn out, and she begrudgingly gave me the mask.

In other parts of the country, hospital staff were creating isolation gowns out of garbage bags. We had meetings on how to improvise alternatives to bleach-based sanitizing wipes. While trying to stay best aligned with PPE recommendations, I was fearful and frustrated. We on the front lines deserved maximal protection. However well-intended the guidelines, the reality of being constantly exposed with limited PPE was chilling. How could we have gone overnight from robust to so ill-prepared, in a country with so much privilege, especially now, when health care demands were only increasing?

Late winter and early spring are always busy times for hospitals. The floors are usually filled with flu patients and those with other wintertime viruses. Yet, as COVID-19 cases started to increase around the city, patients' behavior began to change. Most wanted to leave the hospital as soon as possible. "Please, can you get me home today? I want to be away from here, safe at home," pleaded one patient being treated for congestive heart failure who was not yet ready to be discharged. I listened to her requests and cautiously discharged her by validating her safety concern and committing her to compliancy with her home medications. I knew she was not 100 percent ready to leave the hospital, but I respected her wish not to be exposed.

Wearing goggles, masks and scrubs, I was often looked at apprehensively by patients who would breathe a sigh of relief when I declared, "I am not caring for any patients with coronavirus today." I couldn't blame them. As physicians, we would cohort our COVID patients to one to two doctors to minimize exposure to other patients and keep focused on one area in the hospital. There were days when all I did was care for COVID patients and others when I would not see any. Even so, the pandemic was keenly felt throughout the hospital. I couldn't see the faces of colleagues or patients, visitors were barred, and it all just felt so isolating.

Driving to work started to feel like arriving in a ghost town in the spring of 2020. The hospital parking lots were empty, and hardly anyone walked about campus. Appointments were canceled. Outpatient visits were becoming televisits. People did not want to be near the hospital.

The volume of emergency room patients diminished significantly. The lobby, nearly always bustling, felt serene with so many unoccupied chairs and was permeated by an unfamiliar quiet. Visitors were no longer permitted. Our inpatient hospital census dropped dramatically, even as the weight of responsibility of caring for patients was at an all-time high. On a typical shift, I went from seeing eighteen patients per day in the hospital to ten or eleven every few weeks. The only people admitted were the very sick or those with a bad case of COVID-19. It was eerie, as we expected a surge of COVID patients.

What this was, it turned out, was the calm before the storm that preceded the torrential surges over the following two years.

With the decline in number of hospital patients, pressure was mounting to make adjustments to our staff. Did we have too many doctors on call for a day with not enough patients? We had never been faced with such a conundrum. I began to have uncomfortable conversations on the subject. This was maddening. When we are busy, it's close to impossible to bring in extra help; yet when it's slower, we have to decrease staffing. This is a business, and we are expendable.

It felt insulting and degrading. How could we furlough a frontline physician in the midst of a pandemic? The answer is that finances matter, and with the drop in numbers, the system was stressed. Other health systems across the country were facing similar problems. Colleagues from other multidisciplinary departments were being furloughed, which typically involves a week of unpaid leave and being completely detached from the hospital. I was advised to be proactive.

We made such adjustments as decreasing our staff by one physician per day, a move that was met with disdain. My team was frustrated and so was I, but I emphasized the need for unity, explaining how these adjustments would only be temporary. Certainly our volumes soon would go up, at which point, I predicted, we would get back to "normal"—though I felt like a failure as a leader at this moment. Had I done everything I could have to advocate for frontline physicians—or was I purely a middle manager trying to keep both sides happy? Moreover, was this process sustainable? Anticipating future COVID surges, I questioned if cutting back now would only fail us later, when increased staffing surely would be needed.

* * *

During that first surge in March and April 2020 I felt my life turn upside down. I was jolted from paternity leave into a global pandemic, feeling as if I'd been thrown into a wildfire that couldn't be extinguished. Coming home from work was surreal, driving through empty streets with no traffic; everyone now was homebound. This included our boisterous four-year-old pulled out of preschool as the city was shutting down. Shopping for essentials was an adventure in itself, looking for coveted toilet paper as it flew off the shelves. People were beginning to hoard.

The usual daily grind of parenthood at once became exponentially more challenging. My daughter, who thrives on interaction with her friends, now was stuck at home. Clearly she was frustrated but couldn't readily communicate that, and she required much more time and attention. She was moody and would have meltdowns throughout the day. As boredom set in, even her best-loved activities no longer felt stimulating. Then, what was supposed to be a bonding time between a mother and her new baby turned into Yogita having to both manage an infant and homeschool our daughter at once. Though this was the last thing any of us could have predicted, we joined the rest of the country and locked down for most of spring 2020. We would go for walks, but that was it.

Despite lower total patient volume, the number of COVID patients at my hospital continued to climb over the first several weeks of the pandemic. As anticipated, with recent cuts to staffing, chaos ensued. The burden weighed heavily on me. When I wasn't at the hospital I was glued to my phone, catching up on emails, text messages, and joining online meetings. I obsessively worried that we were on the brink of collapse, too short on staffing and therefore unable to meet patient demands. I was scared we would all become ill.

Online meetings were a double-edged sword. I was torn between two worlds, trying to manage a team from afar and being accessible as a dad at home—where my mind was at the hospital. I felt guilty about wanting to be in two places at once, and I simply couldn't manage it. I could feel stress begin to take its toll. At first, I blamed my constant fatigue on the fact we had a newborn, yet it wasn't just that. The combined stress was affecting my sleep, moods, patience and overall spirit. As happy as I was with our newborn at home, the pandemic and attendant stress took away part of that joy.

On hospital days spent in meetings and caring for patients all day, the question looming largest was, *Am I taking the coronavirus home with me?* My son was only three weeks old, and his immune system was still developing. What if he got COVID?

Yogita and I talked and came up with a plan. I would change out of my scrubs into street clothes at the hospital, to protect against any remnants in the car. (Hospital laundry was done separately.) Then, at home, I would disrobe in the garage and go take a shower before touching anyone. "Close your eyes, Kaiya!" I frequently warned as I ran through our living room essentially half-naked, trying to get to the shower. These changes required our family to make adjustments, which we did. We adapted to the new and strange.

Caring for patients with communicable diseases was not new; I had done it for years and I never took extra precautions beyond the basics. Yet even with these elaborate protocols in place, we worried. Should I isolate myself at home? We couldn't be sure. I had colleagues staying with friends or at hotels, keeping themselves away from their families for days after working in the hospital. For me this was not an option. I refused to separate from my family. I am a father and husband first, and I need my children and my wife.

Even with all the exhaustion and stress, I still felt a sense of exhilaration in those first early months. I was officially part of the pandemic and leading a team of frontline physicians. This was a once-in-a-lifetime opportunity. Colleagues advised me to take a day off, away from anything hospital-related, but I couldn't detach, even when I tried. The drama was (and is) unfolding directly before me and I needed to stay, to be part of whatever happened next. I felt paternal working with my team: I could advocate, navigate, advise and ultimately protect them—a huge responsibility that kept my fire lit during those chaotic first weeks.

Though I always make fun, admittedly I end up watching medical dramas on TV. Whether it's *ER*, *Grey's Anatomy* or any of the others, I like pointing out the inaccuracies and unrealistic scenarios and, often, just seeing the drama. In the first phase of the pandemic, I felt I was watching myself on one of these shows. The days were filled with unpredictable emergencies, curveballs and disaster scenarios. At one point, anticipating a high volume of deaths, the healthcare system provided through rentals a portable refrigerated morgue. Shortages often prompted us to improvise. There was no knowing what might happen next. We were purely reacting to what was being thrown, among grim predictions and complete unknowns, fearful in the moment. We were challenged.

As disaster planning continued, within the walls of the hospital, masking was not yet universally recommended. One afternoon, after recently learning about the need for eye protection, I searched online for goggles for my team and found an industrial-grade style that looked perfect. During the lunch break I ran to Home Depot and found the aisle with protective equipment. To my dismay, I discovered mostly empty shelves and a narrow range of supplies. Clearly, I was not the only one hunting for PPE. Half hidden, though, on the bottom shelf—eureka! A box of exactly what I needed. These goggles were different from the ones I saw online, but they had a high OSHA rating. I threw thirty pairs into my cart and ran to the cashier as though I was part of a relay race and time was running out. Score one for the team. I felt victorious.

During subsequent weeks, my colleagues and I had a small stash of PPE that we kept in our offices, acquired from our homes, from stores or through individual donations. We first had to protect ourselves before we could protect others. We were communal by nature and team players all, but given the risk of depleting PPE, we had to look after ourselves and I encouraged it. I wasn't worried about getting in trouble with administration for procuring and stashing our own limited supply, but I was indeed worried that we well might run out.

I wasn't the only one in our family showing stress. While always super organized—creating a schedule and structure for Kaiya and managing our infant on top of that, in addition to taking care of a busy household—Yogita too sometimes seemed to fray. I would come home and see exhaustion in her eyes. Yet, she never complained. She recognized the crisis we were in. There were days when I worried, going to the hospital, that this simply wasn't fair.

"How are you going to do this all day?" I'd object in near despair. "Kaiya has so much energy, and Kaveh is crying nonstop."

"Don't worry," she'd reassure me, "the worst that can happen is that Kaiya spends the day watching YouTube on the iPad. It is what it is. We got this." (Which is funny, because I am the more lenient as far as screen time.)

Not just reassuring, it felt good to laugh.

One evening, while I was changing my son's diaper, my phone rang. I answered on speakerphone, talking with a colleague about a COVID scenario as Kaveh cried loudly in the background. Yogita came in, offering help and rescue, but I gave her a nod that all was okay. I'd just finished putting a fresh onesie on my son when she smirked and said, "Part of you just loves this. Don't you?"

"Love what?" I questioned.

"This pandemic and everything you're doing."

I looked down at my baby boy while he wriggled and squealed, and I giggled, adamantly shaking my head. The truth was, I *did* enjoy the exhilaration this brought. I truly felt needed and validated at work.

This was historic, and the tone had begun to change as society now deemed healthcare workers *healthcare heroes*. It felt strangely rewarding. There was a global pandemic with suffering, chaos and loss, but part of me was thriving on the adrenaline fueled by crisis. I was leading a frontline team viewed as vital, and we were writing history on the fly, learning day by day about this new disease process, how to treat it, and how to protect ourselves and others. While the world buzzed with the latest COVID news, it was thrilling to be on the inside track, in uncharted territory where whatever happened next was not yet known.

*   *   *

My exhilaration turned out to be short-lived. It started to wane after the second surge in late summer 2020, as we were beginning to see recurrent patterns of the same types of patients. The clinical histories were so similar, with patients having fevers, chills, muscle aches, and getting progressively short of breath. They would try to manage their symptoms at home for five or six days, then frantically present to the hospital when they got worse (which timed exactly to the intense cytokine storm inflammatory response unique to COVID at day seven). All was becoming exhausting and repetitive. We had been in this for almost six months, with no end in sight.

Even worse, it was becoming clear that a portion of the population with COVID-19 simply wasn't taking this pandemic seriously and was avoiding all mitigation measures, such as masking. I was seeing up close what COVID could do, and this behavior was the most frustrating thing to witness. A different portion of the patient population too was at a terrible disadvantage, exposing themselves at work or simply not knowing how to protect against the virus. I witnessed firsthand more African American and Latinx patients admitted for COVID-19 in the second surge. Health equity has always been an issue, and surging in its own way in 2020, I discovered, parallel to what was going on with COVID, was the other pandemic: systemic racism.

Chapter Three

Twin Pandemics

By summer 2020, the second surge was imminent. COVID cases never reached zero and remained steady in the hospital, ranging from ten to fifteen hospitalized patients daily. Other, non–COVID patients were making their way back to the hospital as the summer progressed. We were still in the midst of a global pandemic but felt a slight reprieve, with a lower number of COVID cases for a short time. Predictor models and epidemiologists warned of an impending surge, but it remained unclear to me if and when this would happen.

Thus far my team had survived, and we were feeling more comfortable treating COVID. We also were seeing the more familiar cases come through and populate our inpatient census (i.e., the count of number of patients in the hospital on a given day), which was our normal and, in its way, reassuring. As we approached late summer 2020, though, COVID-19 cases started to tick up—and these cases were increasing much faster. While dramatic, it wasn't as if a switch had been thrown or an alarm bell screamed "SURGE IS HERE" but rather a gradual realization as cases started rising that we were indeed in a second surge.

During this time, on one of my late evening shifts, I admitted ten COVID-19 patients in nine hours. Cases all over the city were going up. (On a typical shift, the average number of patients admitted by one hospitalist can range from eight to ten: these are people too sick to leave the ER—and this time all of mine had COVID.) I felt vulnerable processing this many. I did my part with PPE and my CAPR device but was still left wondering if that was enough. I went home, showered, and went to sleep feeling anxious.

The following morning, I was home and caring for the kids (Yogita had returned to her work schedule). It was 6:45, and our daughter had already crawled into bed next to me. Kaveh was sleeping in the crib nearby.

Suddenly, my wife ran in, scolding me, "Don't get too close to her! Move her to the other side of the bed—you were exposed to so much COVID last night!"

I was cranky, sleep deprived and frustrated. Half-awake, I snapped back, "I wore PPE, and this is the best I can do. *You* stay at home and take care of them if you're so scared of my exposures!"

We both looked at each other and recognized our shared anxieties, fear and exhaustion. Kaiya, nearly asleep, sat up confused and frightened by our conflict. I reassured her everything was okay, and I promised Yogita I would do my best and refrain from kissing them today or get too close. We both knew that would be difficult at best, but fear is irrational and it was plaguing us. And, too, fear of infection became a major stressor in our marriage.

*　*　*

"Sir, my name is Dr. Desai, and I'm going to talk with you about what's going on, as our plan is to admit you to the hospital." This is a basic introduction I present to patients I'm reviewing for admission. This COVID-positive male looked back at me, eyes wide, lips dry and pursed as he took swift and shallow breaths through the oxygen mask.

"No English. Spanish," he gasped.

I responded in Spanish, took his hand (with my gloves on), and tried to give him a vote of confidence through PPE that showed only my eyes. He looked relieved though completely exhausted. He was young, mid-twenties, mildly overweight and had never before been hospitalized. He explained that he worked in a factory and kept on while sick, needing the money.

He hadn't masked or practiced distancing. He became ill five days prior to this visit, having tried Tylenol and some "pills" he got from a community medical office. His breathing got worse, yet he avoided going to the hospital. Now, he reported, he couldn't breathe or catch his breath, and he questioned three times if he would be going on a ventilator. I couldn't lie and tell him no but assured him that we would do whatever we could to avoid it.

Though COVID-19 was unpredictable, I started to develop a gut instinct about whether patients would rapidly recover or get worse. I had an eerie feeling about this man, and thirty-six hours later, he was on a ventilator. To see such a young, otherwise healthy patient decompensate so fast is devastating, but in the latest surge, this was becoming the new norm.

* * *

Soon we began to notice a racial divide among patients admitted with COVID-19. I would glance at our patient list and talk to colleagues, and we saw that the majority of those hospitalized with COVID-19 during the summer 2020 surge were Latinx or African American. At first, the numbers indicating racial disparity among COVID patients appeared to be coincidental, but this trend was sustaining. Without question, COVID-19 was ravaging these minority communities faster, with many getting so sick as to require hospitalization. It was scary. Something had to change.

Trying to determine underlying factors that lead to specific health-related outcomes in disparate communities, especially with regard to a novel virus, is complex and often involves multiple causes. One root problem is that not all were following mitigation strategies. So many were continuing to work and not mask, in jobs that put them in close contact with others for long hours, and these people too were unmasked. Others lived in communal dwellings among extended family, where distancing is all but impossible. And, too, there were those with such poor health literacy that they simply didn't understand what they were supposed to do or why mitigation strategies even mattered.

A lot of these patients had long lengths of stay in the hospital during this second surge. While we were getting better at treating COVID-19, certain underlying diseases made it much harder to treat, in particular obesity and diabetes. A typical patient with severe COVID-19 in this surge would be middle-aged, mildly to moderately obese, with diabetes, and while far too common in my world of internal medicine, these diseases were also far more challenging to treat in COVID patients. Their blood sugars would skyrocket with such high doses of steroids, and the respiratory status of an overweight patient with COVID would worsen so much more quickly.

As in the first wave, these patients rapidly became ill, in ever greater numbers. As before, they typically would arrive on the sixth or seventh day from the onset of symptoms: the peak, we now knew, where risk was highest for progression of disease and morbidity. Younger patients tended to stay home, where they would try every conceivable medication (often including hydroxychloroquine as well as others) until they too arrived with severe shortness of breath. These people were sick and scared. I could see fear on their faces and especially in their eyes; many averted mine entirely, as if there were shame in being sick with COVID.

Sometimes I felt I was outside my body, watching everything happen around me—and I wanted to scream, to plead with myself to *do something*, anything, to stop the spread. There was no controlling this chaos, and absent some action, the sick would just keep coming. Clearly, too, some dedicated advocacy and education was needed for our Spanish-speaking patients. This was urgent. Health literacy— and literacy in general—remains low for so many, and the messaging needed to be about basic mitigation strategies and education around COVID-19.

I joined with a colleague, a native Spanish speaker, to do media outreach to Atlanta's Spanish-speaking population. Our goal was to talk through simple mitigation strategies and emphasize the importance of masking. We also wanted to dispel any myths about COVID-19. We were fortunate to partner with local Spanish media news outlets as well as Atlanta's Latin American Association to do education sessions and Facebook live events. Not only was it rewarding, but it also gave us a voice.

Healthcare workers on the front line of a pandemic have a unique and powerful perspective. Here was an opportunity to be heard. Even if we changed a single perspective, that was meaningful; it was therapeutic, too. Something about the day-to-day grind made it difficult for us to realize the impact of what we were doing. To look outside the hospital walls to share and spread our voices was invaluable.

* * *

While the pandemic was raging around the world, racial injustice was surging here at home. The summer of 2020 was a challenging time for Americans as a society. The murder of George Floyd by police in Minnesota happened in that summer, just as the nation was reacting to the surge. The racial divide in our country was deepening. People were taking to the streets en masse. It was eye-opening and, especially in the midst of a pandemic, scary to see us so divided.

At the hospital, these divisions were keenly felt. Not that any of us were being treated differently; it just felt tense. We were on edge, anxious, angry. Walking into patients' rooms, I would see on TV the videotape of George Floyd being killed, over and over, the wall-to-wall coverage and unfolding repercussions. Many of the protests his murder engendered erupted into violence, and this was happening in downtown Atlanta—and all so fast. What had been a long-simmering problem was now front and center.

I take pride in being patient-centered and advocating for all, yet during this time, I would deliberately try harder with minority patients. I could see terror in their eyes, the lack of insight or any kind of understanding of what was happening. They often lacked ability to advocate for themselves, and it was a true awakening that I could do this for them. I may not have been always successful but I tried. The challenge I faced—the reality—is, what happens once the patient leaves the hospital? Will patients be able to afford their medications, such as insulin? Will they take them as prescribed and follow up with an outpatient physician? These continue to be real concerns.

I made efforts, too, during summer 2020, not only to spend more time educating patients but to communicate with their families, as the hospital remained closed off. While this took much time and added hours to my days, it was worth it.

* * *

"Get out of my room!" screamed an eighty-year-old patient recently admitted with COVID; he was frail, short of breath and confused. Why wouldn't he be? I'd just walked into his quarantined room looking like an alien, wrapped head to toe in a yellow gown, white N95 mask, full face shield and blue head cover. No doubt I'd startled him, but I had no choice. Health workers need to protect themselves at all times when exposed to a highly contagious infectious disease.

"Sir.... I'm here to examine you."

"What?" he shouted, followed instantly by "I don't give a shit!"

I spotted his hearing aids on the side table. All I could think was, *Why hasn't anyone helped put them in? He's going to lose these in the hospital.* Hearing aids are notorious for going missing in the hospital, and they cost hundreds of dollars to replace.

"SIR. DO YOU WANT TO PUT IN YOUR HEARING AIDS SO YOU CAN HEAR ME?"

"No! Go away!" He thrashed at me. Despite my layers of protection, I still felt his claw-like hand on my arm, briskly pushing it away.

Crap! I thought. *How am I going to get anything out of him?* I didn't want to have to come back here a second time only to go through this again. Moreover, to be constantly donning and doffing PPE is exhausting. Sometimes, I would call the patient's phone to check in at some point in the afternoon; but in some cases—like this one—it isn't possible if the patient is confused and agitated. This pandemic had forced me to be strategic about time: I had fifteen *other* COVID patients to see, some in critical or near-critical condition, and much more work to do. I had to keep moving.

"Let me put the oxygen back in your nose, please." I grabbed the clear oxygen tubing that was on the floor and saw that his chest was rising and falling more rapidly than I would have liked. I got the oxygen to his nose under protest, after which I wanted to listen to his lungs, to gauge how much air he was moving. Given this was an isolation room, I searched for the yellow isolation stethoscope—hard to miss, since it looks like a Fisher-Price toy, the kind you'd see in a play doctor's kit. Even so, the stethoscope couldn't be found, no matter how hard I searched. I looked in all the usual places and also the odd spots where it easily blends in: hanging next to the hand sanitizer canister on the wall, for example, or under a pile of tubing and medical apparatus on a side table, or, sometimes, dangling on an IV pole. I searched up and down. It was nowhere. I pushed the call button for the nurse. No one answered. (They all were tied up in other rooms.)

I pushed the call button again, and a voice—not a nurse, but the unit clerk—answered abruptly.

"May I *help* you?"

"It's Dr. Desai, and I need an isolation stethoscope."

"Okay! I will tell the nurse."

I didn't want her to tell the nurse. I simply wanted her to bring me a stethoscope through the door. The patient would look at me and then look away, mumbling and cursing under his breath. I wanted him to be cognizant of where he was and why and that I was not there to harass but to help him. He was upset and likely scared. Hospital quarantine is disorienting. That he couldn't hear what I was telling him only made things worse.

I looked at the white board in the room. The hospital had upgraded these boards to include a section for everyone in the care team's name and a section for family contact. Truth be told, most of the time these boards weren't updated, but I got lucky: a family contact name, identified as his wife.

"Sir," I asked him, "how's Alice doing?"

"I don't know. Where is she? She left me here. When is she coming to take me home?" This man didn't realize how sick he was, and he didn't know that he couldn't have visitors.

"I'm sorry, sir, she won't be able to come. I will call her and see if we can get her on the iPad for you to see her."

"What?! Let me just go home!"

I knew that any further effort to gain his trust and cooperation would be useless. *Still waiting on that stethoscope.* This patient's TV was tuned to conservative news and I was forced to listen to conspiracy theories at too high a volume, which aggravated my nerves. Relief came at last when the stethoscope arrived. Three fast, urgent knocks announced the nurse, who waved at me through the narrow window with box in hand as if it were long-lost hidden treasure. I nodded through my PPE to let her know I saw it.

Then, before I could stop her, she cracked the door an inch or two and, with a flick of the wrist, tossed the box in. It landed on the floor. I felt as though I was in solitary, getting my daily ration.

"Thanks," I muttered, not very gratefully. That door was not supposed to open. Air from a quarantined room must never be allowed to travel outside the room—or so we thought. The stethoscope was still in its package, unassembled. It was like putting Legos together, one piece after another. Not rocket science, but I was frustrated and angry that no one bothered to assemble it. Was I asking too much? (Perhaps I was; the nursing and floor staffing was skeletal that day, as is often the case, and all had jobs to do. There couldn't be time for everything.) I assembled the device, listened to my patient, and observed safety protocol to prepare to leave the room. It wasn't the best exam, but the best I could do under these circumstances. I was, at least, able to hear some air movement in his lungs that wasn't great—not as a result of a poor-quality stethoscope but rather due to COVID.

"I will talk to Alice and see you later," I informed the patient, then immediately washed my hands in hot water and soap for thirty seconds.

Questioning what I really accomplished in that room, I had planned to move on to the next COVID patient (who was alert and conversive and, thankfully, wouldn't fight me) but I still had much to do for the man I just saw. For those patients who are better able to talk and communicate, even with COVID, I would pull up their chart on the computer in the room and talk through blood work, review medications, and place whatever necessary orders. To maintain such a system was imperative, as the COVID patients arrived in waves and I needed to keep close track of their schedules: what day they were on of which medications, along with their lab results. Of course, I had written some of that down on my daily rounding census sheet (a kind of grade list that indicates the patient's "performance" with regard to vital signs, blood work, and response to medications). Yet when fully clothed in PPE, I would leave this document outside the isolation room to avoid contamination. In this case, not only could I not effectively communicate with the elderly and disoriented patient, but he also didn't have a computer in his room. Our goal was to have a computer on wheels in every isolation room, but as the number of COVID patients exceeded supply, many of the rooms were without the needed equipment.

For this patient, I still had to know where he was clinically in terms of medications and blood work. How, then, do I proceed in medical decision-making? I needed to talk to his wife. When should I make time for this? I still had nine more patients to see. I thought about it from her point of view. She's unable to speak to her husband. No doubt she's worried, waiting by the phone for someone to call with an update. That's how my family would be, and that's how I've been in similar situations. The nurses are supposed to help in this regard, contacting families with follow-up information, but again, the workforce was stretched thin and no one had time.

I growled in frustration. In the days before COVID, the family would be at the bedside, where we could talk through things together, and even with patients in non–COVID isolation, I could use my cell phone in their rooms and put the families on speakerphone. Now, with COVID patients, I was just too limited. I kept running into roadblocks. It was maddening.

I knew I had to call this patient's wife right away. I had a sixth sense about it—that she needed to talk to somebody now, and that somebody needed to be me. I didn't question it. I would take fifteen minutes, dissect this case further, and call this man's wife. So I sat down on the isolation floor, N95 mask firmly affixed, and reviewed everything. (I would typically call families by phone from my office, door closed, air purifier on, so I could talk at length without my mask. But not this time.) She answered on the first ring.

"Hi, this is Dr. Desai, the physician taking care of your husband at the hospital." I spoke loudly through the mask.

"Oh, thank heavens! Thank you, thank you! I've been glued to my phone waiting for someone to call...." I could hear her sigh with relief.

"Well, I'm sorry for the delay, but please understand that we are in a chaotic situation, and the hospital is struggling. I promise we have every intention to deliver the best care for your husband, and we're doing that. However, communication may be delayed some, as our staff is constantly tied up and stretched thin." This would become my standard response to the myriad criticisms and complaints about our staff not communicating: a disclaimer that things are not going to be perfect.

"I completely understand and thank *you* so much for doing all that you are doing."

Her pleasant nature and gratitude toward me and our staff, along with a sincere understanding of how severely we were stressed, went a long way with me therapeutically and, in that moment, was exactly what I needed to hear. This phone call was vital to us both. She was compassionate, kind and gentle, precisely how I wish to be with all of my patients. Now, it was she who was providing comfort and reassurance; we calmed each other at a time of great anxiety and frustration.

I gave a clear and concise overview of what was going on with her husband, that he had moderately severe COVID. He required oxygen and was on the right medications, including steroids, about which I explained, "With the good comes the bad. We really need the steroids as an anti-inflammatory for his lungs and body, but there are side effects. We may see more confusion and mood changes in the hospital with him."

"I see. You know he has some memory issues at home, and he's a retired executive who enjoys his life, drinking a few cocktails per night."

Things were becoming clearer. Not only did this patient likely have early dementia, but he was also a daily drinker. I have no judgment against daily alcohol use and would not label anyone an alcoholic. What I do see in the hospital is alcohol withdrawal, which creeps up aggressively in the retired geriatric population, even if the amount consumed is one or two cocktails per night. I explained this clearly to the patient's wife and said that we would treat his confusion as such, that we consider alcohol withdrawal as a possibility in addition to steroids. She understood, and I had to add the disclaimer (as I always do), "This is not to say he's an alcoholic. It's just a phenomenon that occurs in the hospital."

The conversation overall went smoothly, and I felt better knowing that the patient's wife was on board with the current plan. I wasn't overly optimistic, though, about how well this older patient would fare in the next twenty-four hours. He was alone, confused, delirious, dealing with COVID, and getting worse in the hospital.

"Dr. Desai, what can we do? How do I see him? How do I talk to him?"

"Ma'am, do you have symptoms of COVID right now?"

"Yes, I do. It's mild, though, and I haven't even gotten tested. I just assume that I have it."

"Well, that's one reason you would not be allowed in the hospital, as it would not be appropriate to our staff and other patients. And none of our COVID patients can have visitors."

"This is terrible! How can we be in this situation? I saw something this morning, that this may last well into another entire year!" She paused; I could hear her anguish. "I just want this to be over.... I want my husband home. I want to travel with him again. I'll be damned if this is going to be the end of him. I wish the public would understand to mask and follow guidelines...." She sounded desperate for her life to get back to normal.

"I completely understand. What I can offer is to see if the nurses can bring an iPad and coordinate a Zoom or FaceTime visit."

"Oh, that would be wonderful! I don't know how he will respond to that, but at least he can hear me."

"Okay, I will let the nurses know. I will update you tomorrow or sooner if things change. You hang in there and take care of yourself."

We wrapped up our conversation, and at last, I was ready to move on to my next patient. I let the unit clerk and nursing staff know that we needed to try to coordinate a time for this patient's wife to Zoom or FaceTime with her husband. They acknowledged it, and at once I could read their faces: they knew this was the right thing to do, but how would they ever find the time?

"I know this is hard," I admitted. "I'm struggling too. Let's do the best we can together."

The nurses and staff smiled and said, "Okay, thanks."

It helped me, knowing that we were doing this together, pulling for one another, as a team. Even if they didn't need to hear it, I needed to be continuously reassured and reminded that I was not alone—and not isolated—as each new surge brought a further sense of isolation and increased vulnerability. This virus was amping up. I needed the team to support the patients and carry me through the days and nights. Yes, we were all in this together.

* * *

By now, it seemed to most of us that the rest of 2020 and beyond would be spent in isolation or quarantine. Getting together with family and friends in person, as we were finding out, was making too many of us sick. We became more adept at using Skype, FaceTime or Zoom to be with one another, not only to make up for lost time but also to preserve that vital human connection. If lockdown was depriving us of personal contact, we would find another, safer way to communicate.

For me, it's true that all through this time I was surrounded by loved ones at home and at work. Colleagues, clearly, and my team and hospital staff were in close proximity day and night, yet we all were masked and took every precaution, observing every safety protocol. As doctors and professionals on the COVID front line, we had no other choice. At home, as mentioned, my parents lived close by and helped us out daily with childcare. They, too, observed every precaution. Yet, while we were missing every other social interaction, we considered ourselves lucky. So far, at least, none of us had gotten sick, and we were still able to function as a family unit. How many others could say as much?

One afternoon in the summer of 2020, as the country was approaching an impending COVID surge, we were home for the weekend and planned a FaceTime catch-up with my cousin, Smruti, and her husband, Deena, who live in Canada. Smruti is the resilient one, the eternal optimist, who has done so much to help her family through its troubles. My little one, Kaveh, had yet to meet our extended family, and he deserved to be welcomed and shown their love as his sister had in her first year, but this would have to be done virtually, which he didn't understand.

Kaiya, for her part, was running around in the background, waving and poking her face in to say hello.

"Are you at a hotel?" she asked them. Yogita and I looked at each other, confused. Why would Kaiya think so?

"No, Kaiya, we're at home. We're just resting in bed and catching up," Smruti said.

To Kaiya, seeing them FaceTiming from a turned-down bed gave the impression of a hotel room. That they were lying down at two in the afternoon was a little odd, as this was the couple who were always out and about, hiking, walking, being active most of the time. Deena, I noticed, looked exceptionally tired. We knew he had been battling kidney disease and had recently started dialysis. All I could think was, *Oh my God, he looks exhausted—but how do I keep my face from reacting?* Smruti (Kuku, as we called her) was bright-eyed and alert, but it took effort on all our parts not to draw too much attention to his condition. We briefly touched on how he was doing.

"Yeah, Dhaval, I'm hanging in. We're going to dialysis three times per week and getting through it."

"It's harder and harder sitting in that place fully masked for three hours straight," Smruti added. "Everyone around him is sick, too, and they have such strict protocols for me."

I knew exactly what that meant. This was a patient on dialysis going in and out of a hospital unit where he was surrounded by other immunocompromised people in the midst of a pandemic—and all of us were on the verge of another surge.

"We are just trying to stay safe and keep to ourselves."

The conversation turned to other topics, but Yogita and I both sensed that more was going on. Something felt off. Things were not okay. We let the kids be playful in the video chat, and we said our good-byes with lots of smiles and giggles.

After we hung up, I said to Yogita, "Something's wrong. They don't look good."

"What are you talking about? He's on dialysis; he's tired. Nothing wrong with them taking it easy on a Saturday," she assured me.

"I get it, but I feel there's something deeper. They're stressed."

"Probably." Yogita shrugged. "Everyone is, in this pandemic." Downplaying fear was her way of making sure that my mind didn't go to the worst possible place. Besides, as her shrug was clearly meant to imply, I was speculating, based on no more than a video chat.

Even so, I trusted my instinct. Without pursuing it further with Yogita, I grabbed my phone to text my cousin to try to find out more.

Hey, Kuku, thanks for FaceTiming today! The kids loved saying hi to you. Let's talk by phone if you can sometime tomorrow. I want to make sure you're okay! Sorry Deena is feeling so fatigued with dialysis. Let's just chat one on one.

On the screen, I saw the wiggling ellipses indicating she had read my message and was responding. I saw the heart appear under my text, and then *Hey, Dhaval! Sounds good. Yeah, let's chat. How about next Tuesday around 2:30?*

That Tuesday afternoon, I told Yogita that I had a call I needed to take. She assumed it was a work call, and I left it at that (in case Kuku wanted to share something in confidence). Once we were on the phone, I opened up.

"So, tell me, Deena looks really tired. And I can't help but notice your face looked so stressed this weekend. Are you okay?"

She paused. Then sighed. "Yes, I'm stressed. You know I'm strong, Dhaval, and will never let it out. But this is hard ... let me back up and tell you that Deena is so weak. We are fortunate his boss is allowing him to work from home. But between that, the commutes to the hospital for dialysis, and all, we can't catch a break. He's tired. I'm tired. We're isolated."

"I know, it sucks."

"Well, listen to this: we are so lucky that Deena gets to work from home. When his boss first approved this, he had colleagues who had gone to an early summer convention, and all came back positive."

"Oh man, I've heard that story before."

"Yeah, I'm sure you have, and who am I to complain when you're the one that's on the front line bearing the brunt of this all. How are you holding up?"

I saw what she was doing here—throwing the attention back on me. How well I was holding up wasn't the point just now; I really wanted to know what was going on. Part of that is me being a doctor, which comes naturally, even though I wasn't consulted. In such moments, particularly with loved ones, I feel a responsibility to take the lead. After all, if I do this every day with strangers, why wouldn't I do so for my family? (Although, as Yogita likes to remind me, "You don't have to control and oversee everything. Life can go on without you doing that and taking on that burden." She's right, but it's easier said than done.)

"I'm fine, dealing with stress, ups and downs, but handling it." I quickly switched back to Deena. "How is the dialysis situation now? Any alternatives being propo—"

Before I could finish, she cut in. "Hold on, let me tell you. So, since we talked, we have some semi-decent news."

"Oh?"

"You know Deena, with his technical, algorithmic, engineering-type background. Well, he had the foresight to request home dialysis training as soon as he realized that COVID wasn't going anywhere, and it was risky. We've had to go into a hospital each time, and they're full of COVID patients, despite our not being physically in the same unit. So, we've been training, and doing this. It's been stressful, but we got the call that it got approved just two days ago, and we're now expeditiously setting this up."

Knowing how difficult it can be here in the States to set something up as challenging as home dialysis, and how strained in general our healthcare system is, I was shocked and more than a little impressed. That the Canadian health system was able to accomplish this home setup—and during the pandemic, no less—was astonishing.

"Kuku, this is amazing...."

"I know!"

I shared her excitement. "Soon you'll be able to do this in your home. You have the perfect basement for it. You are a very smart person, as is Deena! You can do this!"

"Thanks, Dhaval. You're always encouraging us. I'm scared about it, but we must do it. I will learn and help to navigate it. I don't know how long all this will last. The best-case scenario is that he gets a transplant, but COVID has delayed and messed all of that up!"

"Hmm."

This simple observation made me pause. I knew then that I didn't truly know what it feels like to have a chronic disease and have to deal with the aftermath of COVID in a badly strained healthcare system. Transplants now were regularly delayed and many organs jeopardized, thanks to the virus having infiltrated so many people. So many elective procedures as well were getting canceled due to the overburdened system. A transplant in any case is *very* hard to attain, and here was my cousin-in-law, chronically ill, with a COVID-related delay and complication happening before our eyes. I felt awful for them. Knowing the trajectory of the chronicity of COVID—and this happening in the time before the vaccine—I wasn't optimistic that they'd get the transplant soon.

"What do you think about timing, of when things will return to normal?" Kuku asked. "I feel like we're stuck."

I couldn't sugarcoat any of it. "We *are* stuck. I have no good answers. I'm overwhelmed too. But it's different for me. Yes, it's scary for me to have an infant and four-year-old to care for and protect. But Deena is in a more fragile situation."

"Thank you for understanding."

During our conversation, I learned more about Kuku's fears as well. They weren't imaginary; they were real and not unique to her. I think we all shared them. COVID is scary. I told Kuku that my biggest problem was that I couldn't stay away from social media, especially the headlines with breaking news. It had reached a point that if I looked away for even a few hours, I felt that I was losing control.

She laughed at this (it was good to hear her laugh—something you don't get from texting). "Oh my God! I'm the same way! I need control!

I have to scour every bit of news that comes out about COVID, the possible vaccine, the strains, how to treat it. I know it's doomscrolling sometimes, but if I don't look at it, I just feel out of control."

"Yup."

"And to be honest, I see all these patients on ventilators and I'm so scared of that—I'm so claustrophobic—I don't think I would survive if I ended up on one. If I get it and don't survive, what will happen to Deena in that time? He's sick and needs me, and I need him."

I felt myself choke up. Of course, I'd thought about my own mortality, particularly in the aftermath of a COVID surge, but I somehow still felt distant from it. Perhaps my being on the front line to help prevented such thoughts from weighing me down; besides, it would be too distracting. There isn't any time, in that situation. For Kuku, it felt closer. Her mortality loomed as a threat to her keeping by Deena's side, the two of them alone in their home, at a time when he most needed her. In that sense, it was all about control that could vanish in an instant if she didn't take care. She had to be hypervigilant.

I'm not the person who ever could say, "Don't worry, everything will be okay." Especially now, when we do *not* know that everything will be okay. A false reassurance is no comfort at all when someone's fear is valid.

"I hear you, Kuku. Let's just keep doing everything to protect ourselves and pray." I continue to maintain my faith, and I believe it can be both a powerful and meditative tool for those who share it.

Deena and Kuku did manage to set up hemodialysis at home and avoid those regular triweekly trips to the hospital. It was beautiful, and not so easily done. This isn't simply a matter of bringing in a machine and getting hooked up to it. Dialysis is all about fluid exchange and is rather complex. Their basement had to be configured with special piping and additional apparatus to drain fluid. I was amazed at the pictures and videos Kuku showed me: theirs was a home mini-hospital, with my cousin and her husband doing it all. Kuku had unofficially gained her own certification as a healthcare provider, and by now, she knew more about dialysis than I did.

As the months progressed, we would frequently check in with

each other with updates on our family and whatever else was happening. COVID remained a central concern as Deena continued dialysis. Although they took care not to let anyone into the house, sometimes it couldn't be helped: even their well-oiled dialysis machine had issues, and at one point the basement experienced a leak. They needed to call in a contractor. The moment he left, Kuku had to wipe everything down and spray, to avoid contact with any germs, even from the floors. This was on top of their day jobs. For my cousin and her husband, and countless others facing similar challenges, it was a full-time job just to stay safe.

Yet, even during COVID, life still offered magical moments. That fall, Deena and Kuku received the wonderful news that they had a match for a transplant. The phone call, they knew, was no guarantee; they had been here before, twelve times. With COVID numbers soaring, all could fall through. They didn't stop to tell anyone that night but went straight to the hospital, where the forces were with them. Deena successfully received his transplant, which is a miracle. He has been doing remarkably well. I will never forget Kuku's text the next morning—*Dhaval! It happened last night! Deena got a kidney!* I just looked at that message in awe and couldn't even process it. I was thrilled.

Even as Deena's dialysis ended, I immediately began to worry about their post-transplant lives. Too many viruses and infections, I knew, could destroy a transplant patient, and COVID was certainly no exception to that. Such patients must be careful to maintain distance and take extra precautions whenever they travel, and they need to be especially mindful about whom they choose to be around. Any place that carries risk of exposure, any gathering, even close friends, can be fraught. For a person with a transplant, what was supposed to be the end of complications can feel like the beginning of a new set of risks. Ever the doctor, I'm prone to giving unsolicited advice and information, especially to the people I love. I want them to know exactly what to expect. As I've come to find out, Kuku and Deena are nearly always ahead of me on this.

The truth is that Kuku's stress and fears were real, anxieties that were severely compounded by COVID and everything that followed.

No amount of reassurance, however well-intentioned, can ever successfully quash such fears. I include her story to illustrate a point, that the same is true for millions of us. Our lives have been derailed. In my cousin's case, she did speak to a counselor and credits this with helping her to maintain a certain level of health and positivity. Hers is a tale of survival during COVID with a loved one whose health was compromised and at risk. Theirs was a happy outcome. For too many others, it didn't end well.

* * *

The murder of George Floyd sparked a movement across the country, and with the sense of helplessness came symbolic gestures, most famously, at the time, a kneeling ceremony in memory of Mr. Floyd and recognition of what his death had created.

Our hospital and operations then were focused on the second surge of the pandemic. A colleague, who is African American, brought the idea of the kneeling ceremony to the hospital, that we might participate. As a leader, I was asked how best to proceed. We agreed that the messaging around this would be powerful and give us a sense of unity, and given our staff's diversity, it truly was fitting to do so.

While a hospital-wide kneeling ceremony garnered general support, some felt discomfort, particularly among our leaders. Not that they were against it, but rather, they wondered if the ceremony would create a deeper divide. If certain of our staff chose not to participate (for any reason), might that be used to fuel resentments on both sides? None of this was easy. Any solution to the issue of racism as it pertained to us as we go about our work would take months or years to implement. We had to grow and adapt *together.*

When asked for my view about hosting space for staff to participate in the kneeling ceremony, I reassured both colleagues and hospital administrators that the message would be one of unification and support. The consequences could be worse, I told them, if the hospital did *not* have a space to participate, a point well-received. The plan was approved and the kneeling ceremony took place. It was beautiful, with participation and leadership from physicians, pastoral care, and the hospital. Absent a tangible, easy solution to the problem of systemic racism, our team came together as one, and it felt like a new beginning. In the weeks following the ceremony, initiatives were taken and conversations started around diversity, equity and inclusion that continue even now.

While so many issues remain unsolved when it comes to healthcare inequity and systemic racism, we are moving forward in ways not present before. Even in the midst of a pandemic, the system continues to evolve, along with initiatives, committees, meetings and conversations devoted to these subjects. As change arrives, the most deeply felt will come from the healthcare workers and people on the front lines. After that summer, I am ever aware and reminded that our presence, attitude and ability to advocate will carry patients through their most vulnerable time. Always.

* * *

Systemic racism? some may ask. Let me tell you a story. I'm a Southerner at heart. I'm Indian but also a first generation born in Macon, Georgia. I moved to Atlanta at a young age and went to public school through high school. My friends were diverse. I knew about racism but never experienced it growing up. Living on the outskirts of Macon in a small town called Gray, and then a small suburb outside of Atlanta, I am confident that my brother and I were the only Indian kids at our schools, which included Caucasian, African American, Asian and Hispanic students; few Indians lived in our area at the time. While true that I never felt excluded on account of race, I now question whether I was sheltered in my special group of friends. Was I simply ignoring what was really going on outside of my protected world?

One person with whom I trained during residency in Dayton, Ohio, is my dear friend and colleague Jenny Wariboko, who is African American. We helped carry each other through the darkest days and most grueling shifts with a trust and camaraderie that bonded our friendship. Dayton was not diverse, nor was its healthcare workforce. Jenny would open up and share with me her experiences working as a minority in this professional environment. I saw it firsthand one day as we were waiting on some results for a patient.

"All right, Dr. Desai, I will page you later with the update," relayed an eager nurse.

I was standing next to my colleague, who was also well known on this particular floor. "Dr. Wariboko is here with me and covering for me the rest of the day," I let the nurse know. "And I'm signing out, if you can let her know any updates." My colleague smiled and nodded in a welcoming way.

The nurse acknowledged this. "Okay, Jenny, I will call you later to tell you what's going on."

I didn't think anything more of the exchange. Dr. Wariboko and I had been in residency together for the past few years, and this nurse knew us both on the same professional level: that is, as colleagues, not friends. The expectation, despite our being resident physicians, is that we still be referred to as *Doctor.*

"See that, Dhaval?!" my colleague protested under her breath, so the nurse wouldn't hear as she walked away.

"What are you talking about? See what?"

"You are Dr. Desai, and I am Jenny. Why is that?"

I was silent. I hadn't realized what just happened—right in front of me! The doctor moved on and wanted to continue with the sign-out, but I couldn't move past it.

"Hold on, hold on. Has she done that before, called you *Jenny*? Maybe she just feels extra comfortable and friendly with you, and she doesn't like me as much?" was my response, trying to minimize the situation.

"Dhaval, I'm not friends with her, I've been here just as long as you have, and I have no other relationship with her. I'm Black and a female. She has no desire to refer to me as *Doctor*," Jenny explained, adding that it happens all the time.

I was angry and offered to say something to the nurse.

"Don't bother. It's not worth it. You know how they are. They will make our call nights hell if they don't like us."

Probably true, I thought. "Sorry that happens to you," I said and let it go.

Later that week, it was still stinging me—and with that, an opening of my eyes. I was beginning to see more of what was happening around me. Dr. Wariboko and I had lunch that week, and I had to bring it up again.

"Jenny, you have to talk to me more about what happened the other day. Does the staff frequently do this to you?"

"All the time," she replied. "It's tough being a minority and female physician."

"I had no idea," I admitted. Truthfully, I always knew that women had to work harder, but I'd never before noticed the not-so-subtle derogation, and, to be clear, this was not about ego and pride. Rather, it was about workplace respect and equity. Dr. Wariboko was not being treated equally, and we were equals in that institution, as junior doctors.

"But Jenny.... I'm a minority. I'm Indian. Why don't I get treated differently?"

"Dhaval, you blend in here somehow. I don't know what to say. It's just what it is."

"I look Indian, but I don't sound it, I guess," is how I responded (again, an unconscious defense). I added that it's different for me, being male. "It's not fair to you, and I don't like it. I don't know how to fix it," I told her, perhaps a bit sheepishly, well aware that this doctor didn't expect me to. I was grateful to her at the time (as well as now) for allowing me to see through different eyes.

During those years, I also saw other minority physicians, advertently or not, being treated on a different level. This was ten years before George Floyd and all that happened in 2020 and in a different part of the country. The workforce in healthcare was not diverse, and it was clear that much work remained to be done.

A few years earlier, before summer 2020, a well-respected Muslim physician colleague had one such disturbing encounter with a patient. This doctor, one of the most compassionate and patient-centered that I know, also happens to wear a hijab, in accordance with her faith. One morning, when she entered a patient's room—someone who needed urgent medical attention—she was met with opposition and scorn.

"I want you to go away," the patient declared. "I don't want you here. I wasn't raised with people like you, and I don't want to be treated by you."

My colleague asked the patient if she would be allowed to be seen by her, to help get her through this, and the patient never fully agreed. Despite this, the doctor stabilized the patient and got her through a critical day.

My colleague was disheartened and angry and did not know how to move past this. She came to me as her leader, and together we brought it to the administration. What were we to do in cases such as this, where a hateful attitude based on race prevented a patient from receiving care? The support was there, and while we got some traction around the issue, unfortunately there was no sustained response or plan. This plainly created a precedent, but without formal guidelines, at that time, at least until summer 2020, we were left to fend for ourselves. Today, my colleague speaks on her experiences and is working to be part of the solution. Systemic racism affects not only patients but physicians and hospital staff as well. As healthcare providers we have an obligation to our patients that includes putting a lid on abuse, wherever the source. Today, I'm happy to say, we have a stronger zero tolerance policy. But we're not there yet, as the work, education and training will go on for years around this.

* * *

"Desai? That sounds like an Indian name, but you don't *look* Indian" is something I often hear from patients when they learn my name. The reason, I'm guessing, is that I have vitiligo, an autoimmune skin condition that causes depigmentation (loss of color). Since age nine I've transitioned from a brown-skinned to a white-skinned male.

I've gone through all stages of emotions with this process and arrived at acceptance. Even so, this doesn't mean that I like to be reminded about it. And when that happens, which is several times a month, I begin to question what patients really expect of me—and what I'm expected to look like—with the last name Desai. If they assume I'm Indian, do they expect me to be brown with a foreign accent? Would they treat me any differently or expect a different kind of doctor?

It's caused me to ask questions that don't have clear answers. I never share with them facts about vitiligo but instead brush it off, telling my patients, "I get that a lot. I will take good care of you while you're here."

The events of that summer and the torrent of racism makes me wonder about my vitiligo: specifically, has my Caucasian appearance resulted in me White-passing? If true, have I gained an additional privilege not shared among my African American or Indian colleagues? That certainly isn't fair. Yet what am I to do? I can't change the color of my skin, nor can I cure my vitiligo. Once more I'm reminded that the best I can do is to advocate for my patients and colleagues and use my voice—and continue that work in these unprecedented times.

CHAPTER FOUR

Burnout

I don't have the time or energy for this!

My daughter needed me—right now—to take her outside to ride her bike, and this was my first thought. What *I* needed most was to lie down and close my eyes, if only for a few precious minutes. Outside was sweltering, ninety degrees. It didn't matter. I couldn't say no.

I had come home to a sink full of dishes, the TV on, toys strewn helter-skelter, and nothing put away. "Hey" was all I could manage to my wife as I brusquely moved past her to go change my clothes. I felt tense, angry, frustrated and exhausted. I know she felt that way too.

Kaiya, though, wanted to go outside, so out we went, under a blistering sun. I helped tighten her pink Barbie helmet, and she got on her bike, pushing slowly on the pedals, wobbly and anxious, with me running behind and holding her from the back.

"I'm scared, Daddy!" she squealed as I ran, sweaty and short of breath. Reassuring her, at last I let go, hoping for that magic moment of momentum when, sustained by the pedals, she would maintain her balance and ride free, unencumbered.

"Pedal, pedal!" I yelled—but she wobbled and fell, her own fear preventing her from moving forward. How to get past it, this hesitation and dread, the fear of falling?

We do it again, and we try a little harder.

Watching and helping Kaiya learn to ride a bike does make me proud, yet I failed to feel any joy or excitement. In fact, I was barely smiling, and had to force out a *Yay!* for my daughter. I just wanted to go inside, get evening chores done and move on to whatever was next. In that moment, I catch myself and see that my mood is off, but I can't snap out of it. Instead, I soldier through, trying hard to reassure myself that tomorrow will be better.

* * *

It's summer 2020. We're in the midst of a second surge and the chaos at the hospital is getting worse. Everyone is here at home. Fatigue continues to spread me thin. The past four months are a blur, with no off switch: whether at home or work, I'm always on call. I was overwhelmed, even with full support from my colleagues and leaders, each of whom suggested I take personal time; still, I felt responsible— that problems must be fixed the minute they arise. At the hospital, this meant always. The crises never stopped.

At home, getting rest became a challenge. As much as Kaveh's patterns were improving, I couldn't remember one full night of uninterrupted sleep. I would keep waking up, distraught about work and all the unknowns related to the pandemic: how, for instance, I could protect myself, Yogita and our kids. I was haunted by images of patients short of breath, succumbing to pneumonia and dying on ventilators. Unable to sleep, I would check for emails and end up doomscrolling in the middle of the night, perusing social media for the latest COVID update.

Each day, I'd wake up groggier. I'd start out foggy, then adrenaline would kick in, with the aid of hot coffee or cold soda for added caffeine. My eyes were heavy and my body sluggish.

Before the pandemic, I worked out regularly with a trainer who had become a good friend; now that was gone. I lost weight (muscle mass, mostly) from the stress and not eating proper meals on a schedule. Decent attire, too, seemed a thing of the past: scrubs at the hospital and gym clothes at home, I didn't think much more about it. I told myself the world is in a different place now, chaotic, and that I'm just a part of it—and that one day soon it'll get better.

Self-care, in any case, requires some attention, which can be difficult for physicians and their teams in a pandemic, particularly for those working on the front lines. I clearly saw the risk of burnout and was beginning to experience it myself. I messaged to my colleagues our need to take care not only of ourselves but also of one another. This included all of our teams in all the related disciplines. More than commiseration, this was shared understanding of the dangers of unrelieved and unremitting stress, what to watch out for and what to expect. Stresses ranged from overwork and lack of sleep to the unknowns of a brand-new virus, how to adapt to a world that might shut down, the challenges of homeschooling and related issues, and generally feeling blue. The threat of burnout was real before the pandemic and was now a focus for many. During the first and second COVID surges, I made a point to host wellness sessions for my colleagues to decompress and to always be an open ear and listen. Every one of them participated.

At one such group decompression session, a colleague asked, "Dhaval, you keep telling us to focus on wellness. Tell me, what do you do for your own wellness?"

I was speechless. Fumbling for a response, I could only come up with a tepid-sounding "I do grocery shopping and go to Costco alone," hastily adding, "It relaxes me."

Nobody was convinced. My awkwardness at having been caught off guard certainly didn't help. Some smirked, some smiled, others rolled their eyes.

"You have to do better than that!" one team member shot back. "We depend on you. You're our leader."

There it was: I was doing everything to take care of others but not doing a thing for myself. In that moment, I had nothing more to offer.

* * *

That same summer, Yogita started back at work. All at once, we were forced to make a decision about childcare. In the midst of a second surge, it did not feel safe to send our little ones to daycare or bring anyone from the outside into our home. Caring for and protecting our family unit is our primary responsibility, and that means not taking risks. Kaiya, for instance, could easily bring an illness home to an infant whose immune system was hardly developed. It was decided then that Kaiya would stay home for the summer while things supposedly settled down with COVID-19 numbers. She would join her four-month-old baby brother.

All at once, my safeguard of having Yogita be at home while I was at the hospital vanished, in a flash. Now I was the one at home, managing my administrative world and tending to our kids on my nonclinical days. This meant I needed to work more late-afternoon and night shifts. In between changing diapers, prepping bottles, entertaining my four-year-old and catching my breath, I would be checking emails, making phone calls, text messaging and attending constant online meetings. I was glued to a device, whether laptop or phone, with a napping four-month-old in my lap and a daughter watching YouTube on her iPad.

Days either flew or crept by, some both. We would FaceTime with Yogita in between her patients once or twice a day, which Kaiya loved. "How's Daddy's day going?" Yogita always asked. Most times I would look at her through the phone and shake my head while Kaiya screamed *"Good!"* It was chaotic, and my mind was never in one place at one time.

As the days wore on, I started to feel guilty that I was only half-present at work and at home, shuttling between the two in a state of permanent distraction. When at home, caring for the family, I would question whether I should be at the hospital fielding now constant crises; at the office, I would be torn about where I was needed at home. Each carried its own set of variables, impossible to predict. How was I to know where I should be at any given moment? This frazzled my nerves and often made me impatient, especially with those closest to me. I would text Yogita in the middle of the day, declaring, *That's it, I can't do it anymore. We have to send one of them to daycare.* No sooner would I hit send than I'd be slammed with guilt that I wasn't able to handle it all. It unsettled me.

My parents, who lived nearby, certainly helped. Yogita was working hard, pumping breast milk around the clock, yet she too at times would feel guilty about not being home. My job, though, was to assuage that guilt by showing her that I could do this. There were magical moments, that joy of simply being with my family and being lucky enough to have this time with them, but there were just as many stressful ones when I believed I could no longer do it. In these terrible moments, I felt I was breaking down.

Shared patience became a rare commodity. Often, at night, I'd be resentful about what had been asked of me during the day, considering it "over and above." The house grew tense. I was short-fused with Yogita and would snap at the slightest provocation—the consumption rate of breast milk, for example, or when she would ask how much screen time Kaiya had gotten. I felt I was being grilled. Defensive and annoyed, I would dismissively shoot back, "*You* stay home with them next time!" or "What do you expect me to do?" (The reality was, she did not expect me to do anything more than what I was doing.) Her response to these outbursts only angered me more. Then things would escalate, sometimes into major arguments and meltdowns. I was feeling like a machine and not human, somewhat unseen, and what might best be described as emotionally unavailable. I didn't know what I was looking for. Validation? Gratification? All I knew is that I didn't feel happy. I was going from one thing to another and didn't know how to stop. I was on a high-speed train in the conductor's seat, unable to get off, and feeling as though we were about to derail.

* * *

I was experiencing the all too familiar symptoms of burnout that I had not yet come to fully recognize. More and more, I felt closed off from simple pleasures: those moments with my son, for instance, giving him a bottle. I would look at him and he at me, and somewhere in my brain I knew this time was precious, yet I fought taking it for granted. This is what being permanently distracted can do to you. I didn't have time to appreciate the beauty. Life was moving too fast around me and I was beginning to feel cheated; it didn't feel fair. Our games of "give me a nose"—he would stick his little face out and literally try to touch his nose to mine—started to feel automatic, that I was interacting at a remove. This distressed me no end. Our game had always been one of joy.

Sleep deprivation clearly didn't help, yet how was I to avoid it?

Working late shifts at the hospital is part of the job. Often, I would get home around 1:30 a.m., and after showering, unwinding and crawling into bed, it would almost be time to get up. As soon as I closed my eyes, it seemed, I'd be jolted awake by an energized Kaiya, shaking me and screaming, "Daddy! Let's go downstairs!"

Often, after one of these marathon shifts, Yogita would angrily insist that I not give Kaveh kisses. Her fierce protective instinct was strong, as it should be, but it also could be hurtful. One morning, I snapped.

"This isn't fair to me! He's my son, and I'll give this adorable little boy a kiss or a nose whenever the hell I want!"

Stubborn and angry though I was, I complied. I didn't overdo it with physical affection, and as frustrating as it was, I restrained myself. I already felt like an outsider coming home from long shifts at the hospital. Now I felt like an infectious disease-carrying pariah, having to strip down to my underpants after lengthy exposures and sprint through the house to the shower with dirty scrubs in hand, pitching them into the washer as though they were toxic waste.

Just as stressful were escalating tensions at the hospital—not just for me but for everyone. All the teams were similarly affected, as healthcare was forever being disrupted. While we were busy adjusting to the new demands of COVID and what was happening with our patients, the constant pressure to function as a high-quality team in all other areas never let up. I didn't need a senior administrator to bark and yell at me; I did that to myself. Doctors are trained to not make mistakes and to perform at the highest level, even during chaos. I give myself no corners to cut, which, for me, is the only way to function. That includes needing to resolve or offer some kind of solution for every issue that arises in my group. When a colleague, for instance, is dissatisfied and stressed, I feel a need to remedy the problem. I've spent many an evening glued to the phone, going back and forth with emails and texts on issues I know can wait. But to help in real time gives a sense of control that feels good. During the heady rush of COVID and the second surge, that measure of control kept fueling me.

* * *

Six months into the pandemic and a chaotic home life had begun to take its toll. Soon I saw my worlds colliding, and while these unrelieved stresses and brand-new challenges were initially projected to be short-lived, reality showed me otherwise. We were in for the long haul with COVID. "The new normal" became a universal catchphrase, meaning life as we knew it would be different from now on.

Burnout is real. I could see it begin to take hold in the people around me, not just in team members but others at the hospital, at every level, and with no small dread, I was beginning to sense it in me. My anxiety was high and my mood was spiraling. I was not feeling joy in day-to-day life. I was missing the bliss of seeing my children grow up, of being able to enjoy them and this unplanned time at home. Unparalleled levels of stress, fatigue and untold angst left me in a state of permanent discontent. Telling myself I should be happy, with frequent reminders of all I have to be grateful for, became a strain and a guilty weight. A dark cloud settled over me. It hadn't shifted—refused to—and only became blacker as the weeks and months passed.

Something was going to have to change.

* * *

In the first two COVID-19 surges of 2020, New York City had become an epicenter. We certainly faced challenges in the South with the arrival of COVID, but the situation here was different. The whole country was riveted by what was happening in New York: every day more and more people were dying and hospitals were running out of equipment and space. Case numbers were skyrocketing. Patients were dying in waiting rooms; nursing homes had been decimated; bodies were being transported in freezer trucks and disposed of in mass graves; and the overload was threatening to bring the healthcare system down. It was horrifying—and it felt like a preview of what could happen here in Georgia. How could we handle any further chaos? I was scared, and my mind constantly raced, playing out worst-case scenarios. How to manage a hospital, for instance, if we shifted all our focus and resources to COVID patients. What about the others, those non–COVID patients, in dire need of care? What if we all became infected with the virus, the entire team, at once? Who then would be left to care for our patients? What if my children, my wife and my parents all contracted the coronavirus?

That summer, I first heard of Dr. Lorna Breen from a news article. She was a frontline ER physician and leader, and as I read through the details of her story, everything began to sound familiar. Dr. Breen was someone who wanted to help people and solve problems. She was a trusted leader of her group, had high expectations of herself and her colleagues, and took care of her patients compassionately. It was clear from the article that she strived to be the best and to always do her best. When the first surge struck in spring 2020, she soon contracted COVID herself. She survived without being hospitalized but began to suffer a decline in mental health. Her mental condition grew steadily worse, something she was able to recognize and alert her family to, yet despite their critical intervention, Dr. Breen took her life in April 2020.

This was not the first suicide of a healthcare worker that I'd heard of but certainly the first during the pandemic. Reading her story, I felt gutted. I wanted to pick up the phone, call her, and commiserate. Some part of me realized I needed to talk, but that idea didn't yet fully register. I wanted to tell her that she wasn't alone. I had colleagues who shared her vision and drive, and like Dr. Breen, I too wanted to fix problems and make everything run smoothly as a leader and to provide the best care for my patients. We were alike. The idea of one's own unraveling, of chaos infringing on how I take care of my team and my patients, is anathema. How was I any different?

Reading and reflecting on the life of Dr. Breen, I could feel myself react to it viscerally. I became uncomfortable, nauseous, with tightened muscles and clenched jaw. Dr. Breen could be me or any of my colleagues. This was a tragedy still unfolding.

I shared the article with my group as a wake-up call. From this point forward, we truly had to look after ourselves and one another. My colleagues unanimously agreed. (Two years since her death, Dr.

Breen's family has formed the Lorna Breen Foundation, and President Biden passed the Lorna Breen Act designed to focus on burnout and wellness strategies for healthcare workers. One major goal is to decrease and eliminate the stigma attached to mental health issues (a problem with which health professionals all too often struggle).

* * *

It wasn't until midsummer of 2020 that I fully grasped how much help and personal support I needed. Something more than the usual emotional adjustments (and yes, they include male postpartum blues) that come with the birth of a new baby was happening; I had experienced those before. This felt different. I became more and more short-fused, unable to sleep, and felt not just stressed but oppressed. I was beginning to take things personally. As I went through my day, I was never happy. Yogita recognized it too.

One evening, after the kids were asleep, I sat on the couch with the constant feeling of being drained, without the TV on or phone in hand. Yogita, catching sight of me, asked, "What's wrong?"

I just shook my head, finding it difficult to speak.

"Tell me what you're thinking. I know something's wrong."

"I just don't feel right. Something's not right," I confessed.

"What do you mean?"

"I don't feel happy. I don't feel good. It's more than just being tired and stressed."

Listening intently, she stopped what she was doing and looked me in the eyes. "It's okay to ask for help. Talk to your PCP, and see what they think. I support you all the way for whatever you need."

For the first time ever, I said out loud, "I think I'm going through some type of depression and anxiety."

She nodded. "Mmhmm, and that's okay! You're going through so much, and it's okay to ask for help."

I could neither predict nor foresee the details of that change, and to this day I'm a work in progress, but in that moment, I knew I would have to make a change and talk to someone before I hit rock bottom.

From a career standpoint, this was unnerving. My training as a physician taught me not to show weakness in times of crisis, especially when functioning as a member of a team. Being so affected, I questioned what my advancing depression could imply for my future as a leader. Accepting the diagnosis was difficult enough, but what made it worse was knowing that I couldn't handle this stress. I had made it this far in my career. What was I supposed to do now?

My depression hadn't yet reached the point where I was sleeping all day, shutting down from my loved ones and friends or performing poorly at work. I was still high functioning yet continually exhausted, stressed and lacking all joy. I often thought of Dr. Breen and how easy it would be to slip into a state where the ability to receive help would no longer be possible. I now saw how vulnerable we frontline physicians are—that we all are at genuine risk. I knew I needed to change and so made an appointment with my primary care doctor to discuss next steps.

My PCP knew my history of pre–COVID insomnia and how stressed I could feel on the work front; he also knew how I thrived there. The first thing he asked at my annual physical—after my candid conversation with Yogita—was, "How is your mood?" I let out a sigh.

"How did you know?"

"I've seen you walking around the hospital. I see it on your face. You're struggling. It's time we do something about it."

I never had a healthcare professional tell me I was struggling more directly than he did then. Eyes wide, I was speechless. Choking up, I felt both relieved and seen. My response should've been a quick "Okay, let's do it!" but instead I replied, "Are you sure?" What was it, exactly, that I needed to do? I was hesitant.

He explained and discussed the treatment with me—and, importantly, talked to me as a person, not a doctor. I needed to hear that what I was feeling is common and that there is nothing wrong with starting an antidepressant medication. We talked through the pros and cons of certain medications, and just like that, I accepted a prescription for an antidepressant.

Walking out of his office, I felt instant relief. My shoulders felt lighter, and I was filled with a hope I hadn't felt in some time. Yogita called immediately afterward, offering support. We were in this together. I wasn't going through this alone. I started taking the prescription at night, to help me sleep and boost my appetite.

During those first few weeks, my mood did improve, but another part of me didn't really know what to expect. This wouldn't be a magic cure, I knew, not like antibiotics for a bacterial infection, and certain situational challenges persisted. Yet the medicine was helping me get one foot in front of the other, and I was now moving forward with a lighter outlook on life.

In fall 2021, one year after starting this prescription, I began to feel short-fused again. Stresses threatened to overwhelm me. The pandemic was there, as ever, with the coronavirus constantly mutating against a backdrop of continuous fires to put out on both the home and work fronts. I could handle it, but starting up too was a return of that intense fatigue, feeling of impending burnout, and discontent. I looked into other forms of stress relief, including meditation and the tapping technique. These are very good, well-taught methods but not my ultimate weapons to fully treat what I was going through.

It was during that time, the fall of 2021, that I decided to start seeing a therapist. I was battling a lot of internal dialogue and stress, and my training and experience has taught me that the combination of medications and psychotherapy yields the best result. That fateful decision—to stop internalizing my thoughts and stresses and to seek outside help before it is too late—saved me from the abyss.

*   *   *

While it is validating and comforting to know I'm not alone among my colleagues and peers in seeking psychological support, it is clear that so many of us who might benefit from such help still remain silent. There's a stigma attached to mental health issues, and few in our profession are willing to take that on when it comes to their own mental wellness. Pride, clearly, has a lot to do with it, but pride isn't the only restraining factor. For whatever reason, the brain as it relates to our moods and behaviors isn't seen the same way as are other vital organs in terms of treatment—especially as that relates to the mental health of doctors. There are preconceived notions that a physician, nurse or other healthcare worker may be impaired and not able to function at their best if they are suffering with any mental health issues.

A wise friend in residency once told me, "Listen, honey, we all need therapy at some point." It's true. While I sense some improvement in the healthcare world at accepting the need for mental health support for its workforce, we still have a long way to go.

*   *   *

So now that I am two years into knowing and owning the fact that I must improve my own mental health, how am I doing? The short answer is better. The longer answer, though, is more complicated. Mental health care is not like diabetes or high blood pressure, where you get a medication and start feeling better within three to six months, gaining optimal and sustainable results with compliancy; rather, this is a lifelong journey. Some days are better than others for me, and some situations are better than others.

Before taking the steps that might lead to improvement, I found myself frequently in the dreaded "basement": that dark cold place where my mind would go, often when I'd least expect it. Always, I was ill prepared. I think, perhaps, I'm prone to going there, but somehow managed to compensate, early on, by letting in just enough light to escape the feeling temporarily. School was an excellent distraction, and I kept my mind occupied with other things, too, related to my career. In this I was highly successful, but in hindsight, I see now that the pressing need to be moving on—away from a thought or feeling, perhaps—made me the type who could never sit still. During summers especially, even in high school, I couldn't stand staying at home; looking for a summer job and doing projects around the house were what fueled me. In college, I would pack my schedule with work study jobs and extracurricular activities. I made time, of course, to have fun with friends, but I got anxious if I didn't have something to do or keep my mind busy. As crazy-sounding as it is, it was the only way I knew how to thrive and carry on.

By 2020, it all caught up with me. As soon as our second child was born, COVID struck—and reality turned upside down. No longer could I work the way I used to; our home life was in disarray; the hospital was chaotic and running short on all supplies; patients were dying in rising numbers and every moment felt improvised. Living and leading through what has come to define the times in which we live, it's become crystal clear that what I thought was working well was in fact a recipe for disaster.

Today, not only am I familiar with Dr. Breen's tragedy but also with the cases of other physicians and healthcare professionals who have had their lives completely derailed. I have seen substance abuse, divorce, illness and more among my colleagues. It's sad. We are trained to observe the highest ethical and moral standards and to act in ways that can never be faulted, nor must we ever be found at fault. It really is a pathological way to be groomed into this profession. This is not to imply, though, that my career choice in any way led to a climate of worsening mental health for me. Rather, I believe it was brewing over the course of years, and the double whammy of unexpected work and life stresses at an unprecedented time in our lives simply pushed me to a point where I became oversaturated.

* * *

After starting medication, I did not experience immediate relief with mood symptoms. I did feel, however, a small placebo effect early on—a result of me at long last taking action. I had gotten help and taken the first step toward self-care. After so much resistance, it felt as though a weight had been lifted. A few weeks in, I had a better appetite, and my sleep was definitely improved (not perfect). What I found was that my mind was plummeting a lot less frequently into that dreaded basement. I didn't feel impending doom as severely, even in critical and near-catastrophic situations.

"Dr. Desai, please work with us to get your team ready for this next surge. It's going to be rough. We will need your team's support …" are the type of statements and requests I would hear from other leaders and hospital administration as we prepared for what was coming in winter 2020. I can confidently say that I felt calmer and more comfortable during that period. I was still scared out of my mind about me and my family (especially our Kaveh, who was then eight months old) getting COVID, but I seemed to be processing and accepting it better. I was able to rationalize the doom out of my thoughts, and my moods were, in general, more neutral and even positive.

I was better but not 100 percent. I realized, too, that this would always be true; it's how we process and hopefully come to accept what is happening, without necessarily assuming or projecting the worst, even in the face of real calamity. This process, over time, leads to greater acceptance and a less grim outlook, which improves mental health. I was happier at home and able to genuinely enjoy the time I had with my family. There were also moments of extreme frustration and that feeling of oversaturation. On some days, Yogita and I were at wit's end. Picture walking into a house full of screaming and whining children, the living room and kitchen a mess, and you're exhausted from impossibly long hours, simply drained of energy. Such days and evenings can and do occur. Although medication is for my health, it isn't a fix for the challenges of parenting, marriage, and raising small children in a busy household.

* * *

"What's wrong with you tonight? Something's bothering you. It's obvious," Yogita might ask me, clearly concerned.

Oh no. Not again.

"Nothing's wrong," I would reply, attempting to gloss it over. I wasn't convincing, and she wasn't convinced. All I could ever think at these times is that I'm tired (exhausted, actually), and a big part of me just wanted to say, *Look, it's been a crazy day at the hospital and my patience is low. I'm feeling saturated and my brain is tired. You know I'm on medication to help my moods and all, so I think I just need to sit out tonight—please cut me some slack.* I'd never say that, of course. I couldn't "sit out" for the evening. My kids need their father. My wife needs me to be present. It's only fair.

I needed to fulfill my duties, to fight through this. Yogita worked hard at her new job, even pumping breast milk in between seeing patients, trying to be the best mom she could be. It was tempting for me to use my work toward better mental health as a crutch, to justify that I deserved a break whenever it suited me, according to my mood, but I couldn't. Parenting and marriage don't work like that. It isn't as though I was chronically or physically ill, and Yogita understood, perfectly well. If only my medication could fix the stress and energy drain of parenting! (I know, this is not its intended purpose; even doctors aren't immune from magical thinking.) No, medication couldn't fix what was "wrong"; so much of this tension had to do with the lives Yogita and I created for ourselves. It was never a question of there not being enough support. We deliberately chose not to hire a nanny or arrange for any type of childcare. (Even had we tried, it would have been near impossible during the pandemic.) We did have reliable, ample support from my parents, so we were not entirely alone.

"This is what I signed up for, and I have to do it," Yogita likes to sometimes say, something I often said to her when we first started dating, in residency. I would repeat it when I was in adrenaline mode, to get through whatever the crazy day or week presented. Back then, I had almost none of the cares and responsibilities that I have now. Hers is a gentle and loving reminder not just of where the two of us were but where the four of us are.

The reality was, I couldn't escape the overwhelming daily stress of being at once a father, husband, physician and leader. No amount of medication could fix that, and frankly, part of me was disappointed. I still wanted to be able to do it all. I was trained to do it all. I was trained to not show defeat or make mistakes. I couldn't accept defeat. A wise leader even told me, more than a few times throughout the pandemic, "Don't be afraid to say no and walk away when you need to." Walking away wasn't in my vocabulary. My entire approach to this point had been to keep working, under any circumstance. I had come this far by doing just that is how I would always rationalize it. After all, this is what makes me a doctor, right? Moreover, this is no time to stop. It's my turn now to show that I can lead by example. That means showing that I can persevere through any challenge. I wasn't afraid to show weakness, but the thought of caving to the stress in sight of my peers filled me with unnamable dread. I would certainly be talked about and viewed differently around the hospital and in my professional community—as an example, no doubt, *not* to be followed. Thus far, I had managed to establish my reputation as an attentive, reliable and caring physician. With that comes heightened expectations. In light of any failure, as with all things heightened, it means you have that much farther to fall. To my way of thinking, I would not be *allowed* to say no and walk away without suffering irreparable damage to that hard-won reputation. To do so would appear to be utterly irresponsible. In healthcare leadership culture, there's no walking that back. A fall from such a height only ends in one way: to hit the ground hard and be smashed to pieces. It's wild how high performers keep upping the ante because they simply don't want to fall. So much more is at stake than mere ego. I didn't ever want to hear *We notice your performance has changed. What's going on?* or *This was a shortcoming from you and your team, and we need to correct it,* lest I or any of my team even once be seen as unreliable. As team leader, I will always be protective of our group. Positive feedback and accolades for good performance is what I want them to hear. So if something was to go astray—a complaint from a patient, say, or an unsatisfactory performance—I would take it to heart; that would be on me. I carry that weight and assume responsibility. In any case, the medication didn't change my programming or the ways in which I conduct that part of my life.

* * *

In my annual evaluation with my division director in late 2020, the focus was on the COVID pandemic and how to find the time to broaden my career in light of its heavy demands. In the course of such evaluations, many of us are scared, nervous, and wondering what our job future looks like. I too felt anxious, best described as an eerie butterfly sensation, walking in, but not from fear of losing my job.

Mask on, dressed in navy blue dress pants, a button-down shirt and white coat (I always wear a white coat to meetings at the hospital), I walked into a small conference room with a rectangular table. This was the first time I had dressed up in months, escaping the monotony of pale blue scrubs. The director, also masked and professionally dressed, was seated on one side of the table. As a precaution, I chose to sit on the opposite end (at that time we were socially distancing).

With our manila folders and notepads in place, we began by exchanging pleasantries, then moved to the topic of the COVID pandemic and reflected on the unprecedented challenges. He agreed with many of my points and gave me accolades for leading the team through it all, with a subtle indication (and not so subtle expectation) that we would continue to do the same at the same high level, despite these challenges, in the coming months.

"A hard part for me," I admitted to the director, "is acknowledging that things aren't going to be perfect right now, and operations ... it's like trying to fix the unfixable. We physicians don't always understand that limit. I don't want to let the team down."

Validating my deep concern with understanding, the director reassured me that the team respected me and that my performance was solid; in terms of patient care, he declared that "we won't be able to save everyone" and "we need to take care of each other and understand that." He was right. Our conversation then went in several different directions, and I remember my agenda as not being too organized, though he would always politely defer to me as to what would next be discussed. It's what I imagine a therapy session might feel like. That eerie nervous feeling, however, only grew the more I danced around the subject I felt I truly needed to discuss: the medication I'd started, to help me with depression and anxiety.

I was afraid to bring it out in the open, to lay it on the table, so to speak, before my superior. I knew he'd be the last person likely to retaliate or hold it against me, yet even so, I was downright scared to say it aloud. In our discussion around wellness, I brought up Dr. Breen. Her story was quite fresh at the time, and I shared it with him, as he hadn't yet heard anything about it. As I began to speak, I felt buoyed, almost lifted, as if by a bracing wind, and I woke to the fact that I had no reason to hold back what I was feeling or going through in that meeting with my boss. According to his own words, I was still performing and working well with my team in a difficult, challenging situation; if I were to hide how I felt and what was truly going on with me, wouldn't that only increase the risk of potential harm to myself or to my colleagues?

"So...." I took a breath. "I also want to share with you that I am now taking medication to start helping with depression."

His eyes widened a bit, and he immediately nodded. "Good, Dhaval. We must take care of ourselves."

I smiled and explained how I had gotten to this point. I also told him how much I valued my primary care physician, who helped me thus far on this journey. He wanted more details on how I was doing and if the medicine was helping. I gave him my perspective, and it was freeing to tell him—albeit with the disclaimer that everything I shared with him would be kept in strict confidence. I never believed that he ever posed a threat, but I needed his assurance that our talk on this subject remain confidential.

"I honestly questioned whether I should even share this with you," I awkwardly admitted, smiling. He reassured me that he was glad and proud that I shared and that he would support me in any way he could.

One thing he said has stayed with me. The director concluded our talk by assuring me, "If you ever need to step away from this role for a few weeks or some period of time to take care of yourself, we would understand and support it."

My immediate reaction was, "Thank you, but I'm fine and I need to work." The evaluation ended, and we went on our ways. Yet, once again, I couldn't help but wonder and overanalyze, perhaps, his offer about taking time off if needed. For me, that would constitute a dereliction of duty, an abdication of my responsibility: it's giving in, or even giving up. Still, to this day, I cannot fathom taking medical leave for a condition that I can treat. Indeed, that may change at some unknown point, but I will continue to keep on working, as long as I am able.

CHAPTER FIVE

A Path to Wellness

"Sir, it looks like you're here with COVID and your breathing is affected because the virus has infected your lungs."

This became a routine statement in that third surge, a few weeks before the first vaccine, when cases were beginning to skyrocket. We were about to enter the holidays, days away from Thanksgiving. This patient was a nice, poised and composed Southern gentleman in his seventies. He had come to our hospital from about forty-five miles away, as he had affiliations with other physicians and management of his chronic conditions in this area. As I reviewed all of his blood work, X-rays and history, he shared that his wife was home with COVID but doing okay. He was frustrated, explaining that he "did everything to avoid it" and was "extra careful."

Recognizing and validating his frustration and concern, I reassured him that we would get him through this and explained the entire care plan, with which he fully agreed. I was used to patients second-guessing remdesivir (if they needed it) and its side effects. He said he trusted us and thanked us for the great work and care. Knowing that he came to our institution with trust and respect was refreshing, and especially that he would not impede any progress with resistance or presumptive ideas about medications (such as ivermectin or hydroxychloroquine, which don't work). I let him know that I wouldn't be able to see him the following day (I was working a late shift) and that one of my colleagues would be assuming his care in the morning. This COVID patient was one of many I'd admitted that day, all with varying degrees of respiratory issues and illness.

A few days later, when I was back on rounding (caring for patients) on the day shift, I saw this man's name on my list. I immediately recognized it but couldn't remember details of his clinical condition or what he looked like. As soon as I glanced at the chart, however, and reviewed the specifics about his case, it became clear which patient this was. (With such a large turnover, one of the downsides of working in a hospital is that we don't have enough time to establish meaningful relationships, so names and faces are often hard to remember. Reading notes and specific documentation nearly always helps.)

I was happy to see him, to be able to connect and have that continuity. Best of all, he was looking medically stable, enough to be discharged that day. Getting a COVID patient in this person's age group out of the hospital is special, every time. At the start of the pandemic and through the first and second surge, our hospital would make a "Code Rocky" announcement whenever a COVID patient was discharged. (Here referring to the character Rocky in the movie, who perseveres and emerges the winner against all odds.) The entire staff would erupt in cheers and gather in a line out front, exuberant and waving and shouting *Hooray!* as the patient exited the hospital. We all would get excited and be thrilled to participate. Yet, by the third surge, these "Code Rocky" celebrations were few and far between; too many COVID cases were piling up, with patients coming and going all day, and no one had enough time to dedicate even a few extra minutes. To me, it was still and always will be a special occasion to be able to discharge such patients.

When I entered this patient's room, he looked tired but still was smiling and conversive. He appeared to be the kind of person who took care of himself, clean-shaven, well-dressed, but now was disheveled. I asked his permission to do a physical exam, after which it was clear that he was ready to go home. (Often, such patients who are ready to be discharged tell us that, in fact, they don't feel ready and are "too exhausted.") This patient was different and told me, "Okay, great!" when we talked about his going home. I wanted to make sure that his family was in agreement, as his wife was still at home with COVID. Both would be there alone.

"Sir, can we put your family on speakerphone?" I wheeled the computer over to his bed. I was fully gowned, wearing goggles, and speaking loudly through a mask strapped tightly around my head. I felt as though I were yelling, but he seemed fine with it.

"Sure, hold on one minute...." He grabbed his cell and started going through his contacts, then dialed.

I saw his wife's number on the white dry-erase board but couldn't get my cell phone out to call. (I was gloved and in an isolation room.)

It rang several times. I was hopeful that someone would answer. I didn't want the call to go to voicemail, as often happens when a family member is needed.

"Hello there!"

Hooray! His wife picked up.

"The doctor's in here talking about me going home. Talk to Dr. Desai."

"Okay. Hi, Dr. Desai, let me connect on conference call with my daughter," explained his wife. I was fine with waiting. It's best—and most efficient—to get all questions and concerns addressed at once, when the family is together.

Once their daughter came on the line, we talked as a group about how the patient was progressing, and I stated how impressed I was by his improvement. They were thrilled that he was coming home. After reviewing his medications (what was given while in the hospital, what we were stopping and those he would continue on discharge), I checked the pharmacy name and sent his prescriptions and paperwork electronically. The pharmacy was able to do home delivery, which was a blessing at a time when the couple couldn't get around. They were grateful for me and remembered my name from the day he was admitted.

"It's the best feeling, knowing I can discharge someone I admitted," I avowed. "I'm so happy you're going home." Then I added, "You're still going to feel like you were hit by a truck, and the fatigue will be there. The best thing you can focus on is hydration, getting enough calories in you, and continuing to quarantine." I also explained that after their quarantine, they should continue to mask in public and follow all mitigation measures.

"Doctor," they were quick to respond, "we've been patients in the healthcare world for years, along with family members. We think we should all be masking." Their demeanor and well-informed response were refreshing.

While not thrilled with the idea that they couldn't yet see family, they understood the necessity of quarantine. Here were two empty-nesters in need of support to help them get through this last stage of illness—and still, they assured me, "We'll be fine and get through it. Family and friends will drop off meals to our door."

Discharge orders went in, and I shared with them my contact information. I would be there for help if anything came up.

Two days later—it was a Sunday afternoon—I was wrapping up for the day before heading home, after starting very early that morning. (I always like to start extra early on weekends so I can be home as early as possible to be with the family.) As I was cleaning up my electronic medical record inbox, where I sign off on notes and orders that were pending signatures, something just wasn't sitting right. I came across this gentleman's discharge summary from that Friday. I recognized the patient's name and clicked on it.

First, I checked the record to make sure I didn't see any hospital or ER visits across the system after I sent him home (which is the worst, finding out that a patient I sent home is back in the ER or has been admitted only days after being released from the hospital). After I read through this patient's discharge summary, checking for any errors or additions, I signed off. I still had an eerie gut feeling about him, though, so I called his home.

His wife answered. Her voice was hoarse and she sounded fatigued. "Oh, thank you so much for calling. He's napping right now, doing okay, but not eating much, slowly getting energy back, and we are alone quarantining and haven't seen family. We will wait to see our primary care physicians for follow-up."

As she relayed and explained all this to me, I understood that they were following the quarantine rule, observing safety protocols and being compliant. With that, I could sense the isolation and loneliness in her voice. I felt sorry for them and began to worry about what my parents would do in a similar situation, if they were in quarantine, alone and sick.

I had a good feeling that this patient and his wife would recover, but I decided to give her my cell phone number just in case, as both were in their seventies and still at risk. I always trust my instinct when a risk may be involved for a patient or the family. She wrote down my cell number and promised she wouldn't use it unless something urgent came up. To be clear, I rarely give patients my cell phone number, and those few times when I have done so, it's only been utilized in extreme circumstances.

Three days later, during the week of Thanksgiving, I was working at home when my phone dinged. I was in the middle of a Zoom call on my iPad, with Kaveh in my lap getting a bottle. I glanced at my phone and saw a text from an unknown number.

Dr. Desai. This is Mrs. G. Our daughter E (40 years old) is coming via ambulance to ESJH ER from Roswell with bad COVID. Please help her. We have already lost one daughter and twin granddaughters at birth. Please.

My heart sank. The feeling of urgency and desperation here was palpable. I knew that I had to help, but what could I really do? During an outbreak of COVID in the midst of a surge, the hospital system is severely overburdened, and there is hardly a way to rush or prioritize one patient over another.

I responded by text that I was not at the hospital but would pass the name along to the ER team in case her daughter got admitted. In that moment, it was the best I could do—to give at least some reassurance when she was not only scared but feeling helpless, alone and stuck at home. Even had she been able to travel, she wouldn't have been allowed into the hospital, which would have increased her panic. By being there for her, if only by a text, I was able to deescalate some of that fear—that lack of control that families feel in an emergency, when the lives of loved ones are at stake.

I later learned that her daughter had chronic medical issues that included asthma, and she was so short of breath, with difficulty breathing, that she came straight to the ER that was full and saturated with patients. Fortunately, she arrived later in the morning, so the patient load was *slightly* less. Unfortunately, she was sick enough to be admitted and was given a diagnosis of COVID pneumonia that required that she be put on oxygen.

Fast-forward three days. I'm back on clinical service to work the holiday, and E (daughter of Mr. and Mrs. G), coincidentally, is on my patient list. I trust my team, so I didn't feel the need to micromanage her admission and details. In fact, I hadn't even glanced at her chart. Also, I hadn't heard back from this patient's family, so all was likely moving in the right direction.

She was a younger COVID patient (at forty) but still so symptomatic and sick. She was weak, short of breath and feeling miserable, as though she'd been hit by a tractor trailer. E is a high school teacher and extremely social and active, making confinement in isolation that much more difficult. As soon as I introduced myself, she knew exactly who I was. In the space of seven days, I had gotten to know this entire family through COVID. E would open up and share with me what she noticed about our hospital staff, how stressed they all were, and we talked about shortcomings. I described the unprecedented challenges of what we presently faced as an institution and shared that there were issues and that we were doing the best we could under these extraordinary circumstances. She completely understood.

While I worked with E and navigated her care, we would regularly check in with her parents via speakerphone. Those calls provided tremendous relief. They could hear her improving day by day, confident that she would soon get to go home. My perspective now is considerably different from what it was before I became a parent. I well understand that hopeless, helpless feeling when a child gets sick and there's no easy remedy, no quick way to make them better. The parent is consumed with a worry that won't stop until the child shows some sign of improvement. Then and only then do the fears abate. In this case, both parents trusted me and the medical team, which went a long way to help ease their anxiety.

Soon enough, E was able to go home and had my cell phone number just in case, as did the family. Her recovery from COVID went smoothly, and she got back to teaching after taking some needed time off. After I'd written her school a note to authorize her leave, I knew what a valued teacher she was when her principal wrote back, *Dr. Desai, please tell her to take her time. We love her and need her back when she's ready.*

*   *   *

Two weeks after this family's daughter left the hospital, I received the following text: *Hi, Dr. Desai! This is E. You treated me and my dad a couple of weeks ago. First: thank you. My medical history has made me a connoisseur of medical care. You and your colleagues provided unparalleled care, emotionally and physically. When I was septic in high school, I kicked a neurologist out of my ICU room and off my case. My primary care physician said, "but he's the best at what he does!" I told him to find the second best because I don't care how smart he is if he's not kind! You are both.*

Several weeks after that, she checked in with me again to say, *Just want you to know that I am praying for you, your colleagues and patients. Thank you for being a light for so many in this dark time. On the first day of school last week, one of my students said he wanted to shake the hand of the person who made me better but he'd wait until COVID was over!*

Here was a case of an entire family who had suffered with COVID, which at that time was not at all uncommon, with whom I'd been able to connect. I could see up close how their lives had been affected, what they were going through, how much was at stake. These were not just patients X, Y and Z being shuttled on a gurney into isolation rooms, to be processed in an anonymous, faceless system. It was my face behind all the masking and goggles, my sharing of hope with them and caring about what happens, which is also to say that healthcare is a two-way street. This family was one of many at a time when vaccines had not yet arrived, cases were exponentially rising and society had started experiencing pandemic fatigue. When reflecting on that now, and with this particular family (as well as others), I truly feel grateful that I was able to help—first and foremost, that they recovered from COVID and our care team got them through it. This was during the third COVID surge, by far the worst for healthcare workers; with such patients and others like them, it was a reminder that we were actually making a difference. By that point, we had all but ceased hearing the same positive feedback we did at the start of the pandemic.

Thankfully, the universe brought me into contact with this family at a time when I needed it most. I had been dealing with stress, mental health issues, burnout and fatigue; that all-important validation, so necessary in moments such as these, can be elusive. What happened at this time with this family for me was a reminder that the small things we are able to do—a simple kindness, in this case—can have such a meaningful impact. I knew then, too, that the compassion shown back to us is equally as gratifying, and it truly fueled and motivated me when my energy and morale was lowest. The concept and feeling of gratitude are vital to physical and emotional well-being. Amid chaos, stress, and just trying to survive, I was struck by how much I needed to be grateful, not simply for my life but also for all that I have in this profession and, most importantly, for the privilege to care for my patients. It's more than a job and career. Being there for the patient is my primary responsibility, one that, with hope, continues to bring me joy.

* * *

From the standpoint of my mood and mental health, the periodic surges from 2020 to the latter part of 2021 and early 2022 formed a pattern of peaks and troughs. The peaks were those intense, long days and nights when we were inundated with a high number of sick patients to care for and an exhausted, overworked workforce. The troughs weren't really troughs in the usual sense, where the pace is calmer and more laid back, but rather troughs in the hospital's COVID numbers.

After being on medication for about a year, I felt that the improvement in my moods had plateaued. Crankiness returned, as did my short fuse. Energy levels were adversely affected, and my sleep again had become disturbed. More and more, I found my mind going to the basement, along with the feeling of doom and dread—and, frankly, of being overwhelmed again. I was angrier and more frustrated.

At home, my daily duties and interactions were a burden. If I had to adjust my schedule (which was far more flexible than Yogita's) for any reason—to make sure the children were picked up, for example, or if something had to be done around the house—it made me bitter. That bitterness soon turned to resentment. I was doing everything, I'd tell myself, which couldn't have been further from the truth. No matter. It was tunnel vision, and a dark tunnel at that, which had begun to feel harder and harder to escape.

The blowouts and arguments with Yogita had decreased but continued to happen, and many would occur at those times when I was feeling the lowest, without my even recognizing it. The meltdowns were often over something silly (but certainly didn't feel so at the time). I also remember being short with my parents over ordinary questions or simple suggestions. I just didn't want to hear it or get involved in conversation. This was probably my body's way of telling me, *Dhaval, you need to slow down. You're hitting rock bottom fast.*

* * *

All through medical training, we are taught the best and most effective ways to treat specific conditions, including those related to mental health. For depression and anxiety, for instance, medication and psychotherapy is recommended. In my case, I had always been open to the idea of a therapist but never truly wanted to connect with or commit to one. I'd spoken briefly to some workplace counselors over the years who were available to us at the hospital. As helpful as they were, I knew at the time that these were short-term fixes and that I needed to establish something longer-term, where I could delve deeper and develop a relationship. I knew as well that I had to get back to exercising, as that had all but stopped. The pandemic was the perfect excuse to cancel sessions with my personal trainer and stop going to a group fitness class.

One night, I just declared it outright to Yogita. "It's time I think I want to talk to a therapist." This wasn't up for discussion.

"I think it's a great idea, but you have to promise me you're going to stick with it."

Yogita well knew my decision to commit could easily turn into "feel better, move on." We both knew this big step had to be longitudinal.

I assured her that my feelings about therapy had changed, that I was no longer ambivalent and that I was ready. Moreover, I was able to find a therapist locally, referred by a trusted friend one day while we were having lunch. I happened to open up about challenges, which must have resonated, because then he opened up, sharing with me the name of his therapist. After our conversation and my friend's enthusiastic referral, I decided that I could be helped too.

The stars aligned, and I must've been at the right place at the right time because this therapist turned out to be just the right fit.

To be able to decompress in a professional setting and to talk about any issues, big or small, has been not only therapeutic but also refreshing. As Dr. Breen's story shows, people in my field can be loath to seek help due to fear of the stigma believed to be attached to psychiatric illness. The reality is, that if left untreated, poor mental health can lead to a devastating outcome. In my case, my fear was not that of being labeled but rather of being seen as someone who was struggling and unable to handle whatever was coming next—in this instance, a COVID surge. My Type A personality thrives on such challenges and all the stresses they entail; what I needed help with was to learn how to take them on in a healthier manner.

One of the most gratifying aspects of the therapeutic relationship is that my therapist is not all about comforting me or providing reassurance that my decisions are correct. Rather, he challenges me to look at things from different angles and to consider myself when making certain choices. It's been pointed out, for instance, that I'm in a high-functioning part of my life and wearing too many hats. He wants me to find a way to keep doing that but know when to stop and say, *It's time I find a few minutes of my own. I'm feeling saturated.* That's where I always fail. I never know when to stop until it's too late. At first, I thought I would feel angry at being challenged or asked to change myself; the truth is, challenging me on how I come to certain decisions is the most useful thing that's happened.

My relationship with my therapist is ongoing. We meet on average at least twice a month. He has given me homework, to journal what is happening when my mind goes into the gutter and why. We have uncovered themes of dread and more. All in all, so far, this has been very effective.

* * *

In fall 2021, I made another change. I committed to a regular physical workout with my friend and personal trainer (we were both vaccinated and his private studio is ideal for the workout). Before the pandemic, I was getting routine exercise and attending his group fitness class. That cardio and strength training provided a benefit that, well into the pandemic, was sorely missed. I was getting no physical release from the combined and compounding stresses of work and home life, no way to decompress. Now, with the vaccinations and boosters, I felt safe working out with someone one-on-one. It's a great way to decompress and escape for an hour (from urgent emails, texts, and all things related to home and work). Just as my therapist offers me challenges, my trainer challenges me on a physical level, to push myself to various extremes, and that in itself brings on natural endorphins and a deep feeling of gratification.

* * *

Moving into late 2021, helped by vaccinations, work began to settle into more of a routine. From a COVID standpoint, we were starting to wind down on the Delta variant, with fewer hospitalized COVID patients. I, too, was starting to feel more settled. Although my therapist, a psychologist, doesn't manage medications, he has experience with their use and effectiveness among his clients. As he got to know me better, he made an important recommendation: sometimes, he said, it's a matter of trying a medication along with therapy. Maybe the medication I was using wasn't providing the benefit I needed. While I was seeing partly cloudy skies with occasional sun, how do we get to the mostly sunny skies on more days out of the year?

On a crisp and colorful late autumn day, I'd just finished an intense workout, having pushed myself that one last bit to a feeling of fatigue and euphoria. I felt clear and was enjoying the benefit of exercise, well knowing that this feeling wouldn't last. This fleeting sense—to be filled with a strength I don't always feel and that everything is truly okay—is all the more precious (and also a bit puzzling) as soon as it departs. I would try to make this a part of my weekly routine (a complete daily workout isn't possible). Driving home, I put on some of my favorite music from the 1990s and early 2000s and started feeling nostalgic. It came as a kind of epiphany, then, when I realized that I was doing everything I could to care for myself. I was meditating, exercising, taking medication and going to therapy, putting in the effort to improve, but I wasn't there, performing in that optimal, superior space. The problem is what it always is, that I set expectations to a point beyond reach. The standards of performance I hold for myself are nonnegotiable, and I'm challenged to accept anything less, even if it's the right thing to do.

"I think I should talk to my PCP about maybe changing medication for me." I explained this to Yogita in a defeated tone and, admittedly, feeling deflated. I felt as though I was disappointing us both.

"Do it. It's fine. I have patients that I treat whose medications change frequently. It's not a big deal," she reassured me.

Part of me wanted (and, therefore, expected) her to say, *No, this is enough. Let's not do anything more and focus on something else.* I was quietly looking for a way, with her support, to keep my mood changes on the back burner and not let this issue become too big a distraction. Yogita is smarter than that, and in this instance, she was one step ahead of me.

"Are you sure you're okay with that and will support me?" I questioned.

"Why are you even asking me that? Of course, I'm your wife. Text your PCP now and set something up."

I did that and set up an appointment the following week.

The last thing I wanted to do was to make my mental health a central focus or one that takes time and energy away from my family because it needs ongoing management. Instead, like most people, I wanted a quick fix so I could get back to my life. Yet, on that particular afternoon, listening to music on the drive home, it was a culmination of things that hit me. Wellness is more than just a route to follow; it's one's own path, and I'm the ultimate conductor on the train for this challenging ride. There will be torrential storms, delays and sudden stops that will lead me to shift gears, change direction, do what I need to, to avoid burning out, crashing or derailing. Medicine, after all, always had been touted as lifelong learning; why wouldn't I transpose that same practice into my life and apply it to my own lifelong trek?

* * *

My PCP and I both agreed to the change in medication. I would need to begin tapering off the old prescription—that is, decreasing the dose by certain milligrams and a certain frequency, at the same time slowly starting the new medication. Sounds easy, right? Wrong! This process, which took two to three weeks, was the most challenging for me ever, physically and emotionally. I was ready to make the change, but even as an experienced physician, I had no idea what I was about to experience.

Lying in bed that first evening, about thirty minutes after decreasing my dose, I closed my eyes and the bedroom started to spin. I felt wildly unsteady, as though I were on a roller coaster.

"I feel dizzy," I said, alarmed, waking up Yogita.

"Maybe your blood sugar is low? We ate dinner early. Do you want me to get you something?"

"No, let me try some water, and let's see what happens." I grabbed a glass of water from my nightstand, took a few large sips, and the dizziness gradually subsided. I laid back down and, at last, I fell asleep.

The following morning and for the next few days, I felt a weird foggy sensation, not of being drowsy but rather cloudiness, incipient headache, and an overall feeling of just being "off." Yogita and I both being physicians, we instantly suspected the worst. COVID, we knew, sometimes shows up with nonspecific symptoms, and given that I was vaccinated, we wondered if this well might be a mild case. Home testing had just begun, and thankfully, I tested negative. If not COVID, then, what could be causing the dizzy spells, headaches, fogginess, overall lousy feeling? We remained in the dark and it didn't take long before our minds went down the rabbit hole.

The next several nights, I would lie in bed and feel as though I was racing up and down a hill. It was bizarre and scary. One morning, Yogita woke in tears, beside herself with worry. Usually, I'm the one overwhelmed with anxiety and imagining the worst-case scenarios; this time, it was Yogita, which doubly frightened me. Both of us were thinking *brain tumor*. All the symptoms fit. We had seen many patients suffer through it.

We soon came to our senses and decided that the likeliest cause of my ongoing symptoms must be related to the change in dosage as I was tapering off the old medication. We hadn't considered it because we hadn't been aware that this could happen. We did our research and concluded that it was indeed the medication change. The dizzy spells were the worst. They would come at once, sometimes when I was driving. That was scary.

Just when we thought the side effects at last had subsided, it was time to start the new medicine. That was the plan, and I would follow it. Nothing could have prepared me for the nausea that ensued the moment I started the new prescription. The dizziness was gone, but the nausea was unlike any I'd ever felt. It was deep in the pit of my stomach, not the usual kind that I get when I'm about to vomit. This was a nausea mixed with butterflies, such as those brought on by nerves. It was constant and unrelenting. It was uncomfortable. Anti-nausea medications did help some, but I didn't want to have to take them all the time. I was reassured by my PCP that gastrointestinal side effects are common at the start of this particular drug (likely from all of the serotonin). I didn't want to accept this explanation. I simply wanted the nausea to end.

One afternoon, before working a late shift, I was lying down in our bed. Yogita had picked up Kaiya earlier in the day and brought her home. They were still downstairs. I felt physically miserable and couldn't nap. I knew I had to go to work. I called to Yogita and asked her to come upstairs, alone. I didn't want Kaiya to see me in this dreadful state. When Yogita entered, I broke down in tears. I told her that

I felt like crap, that this constant nausea and attendant feeling was too hard. She understood and recognized all of this as related to the medication. She suggested, as one possibility, that we go back to the old medication and stick to that. My response was that I didn't necessarily want to give up, which meant stopping after coming this far. She didn't discount what I was feeling and once again reminded me it was the medication; she had seen her patients experience similar side effects. I decided to march through it.

Two days later, still afflicted with nausea and anxiety, my emotions went haywire. I believe it was my body adjusting to the new amount of serotonin flooding my bloodstream and brain. Serotonin is a hormone that affects all parts of the body, and this is to be expected; nevertheless, I had reached the point where I could no longer fake what was truly going on with me. I couldn't pretend to enjoy the company of my family, on a lazy Sunday morning like this one, for instance, while these unremitting symptoms threatened to take me down. I bolted, literally—I ran to the bathroom and sobbed while dry-heaving, and this went on for some time. That, thank God, was the worst of it. After a few painful days, my body finally did adjust, and I started to feel much better. It was a very rough transition from one medication to another, but I needed it.

As the foregoing makes clear, we all—even doctors—need to educate ourselves about the uses and effects of prescribed medications, especially when starting on a new one. Without going into specific names or brands (I don't wish to discourage anyone or steer people away from a prescription they might well need), I do wish to emphasize that if you're experiencing side effects, speak with your doctor. Having gone through this myself, I am now more aware of what can happen when a medication is changed and of the need to talk through possible side effects with my patients moving forward. I've learned that being a patient and going through what patients do, and what their families go through as well, is the best way to become a better doctor. This is the truest, maybe even the only, way to relate and fully empathize.

* * *

A few months into the new medication and adjustment with therapy, I felt I was on a much better track. This leg of the trek was much smoother. Yogita's primary concern was that I keep the focus and continue to work through things and not give up on therapy. She understands how vital it is for my health and that I have that important outlet. As she well knows, it is all too easy for me to move on, especially when I'm feeling so much better. She supports me and wants to make sure that I stay on the path. I respect and appreciate that. To this day, I keep up with both medication and therapy. I'm having many more good days than bad, and, so far, I continue to improve.

* * *

"Dhaval, may I talk to you for a few minutes today?" asked a close colleague from another department.

"Sure, let's set up a time this afternoon." I figured we were going to talk about hospital and related matters. Later that afternoon, between busy rounds and meetings, I barely had time to meet but didn't want to cancel. As my colleague came into the room, she closed the door. We started with pleasant chitchat, mixed with a little hospital gossip. (Television, after all, doesn't have a monopoly on medical dramas and soap operas.) After a few moments of catching up, she suddenly became serious.

"I'm just sick of this and burnt out," she confessed.

"What do you mean, *burnt out*? I feel like we use that term too sparingly."

"I'm just not happy."

"At work or at home?"

Pausing to think, she replied almost reluctantly, saying, "Well, all of it, if you really want to know." I nodded, and she continued. "I'm forty-three and constantly *on* and busy with my career and home life. I have a supportive spouse and all. My kids are young and so needy. None of this is bringing me joy. I don't know what to do." That's when the tears started.

I was quiet and listened. I validated. "Is this the first time you've felt like this?"

"I don't know, it's been like this a few times, but never this bad."

I could see it all in her eyes. She was miserable. For her to come to me, a person who wasn't even a very close friend, was alarming. I'm glad she chose me as her confidant, though I was worried.

"You know, I'm going to share something with you, and maybe it will help, but I want to ask you first. Have you considered that you may be going through depression?"

"Of course I've thought about that. I'm a physician, and we diagnose ourselves. I've been too reluctant to do anything about it. I don't even know where to begin. And I'm scared to really admit it, as I do have good days ... and it all just feels like maybe it's the part of life I'm in and I just need to overcome it. This pandemic and treating all of these COVID patients has taken a toll." I nodded.

"No one knows this, and I'm going to share it with you. I was going through similar things, and I know it may feel like a different perspective because I'm a male ... but I'm on an antidepressant and also seeing a therapist."

Her eyes widened in surprise. "You?!" she exclaimed. "Come on. Are you kidding me? You—always smiling, and *so* on top of your game. I've seen your Facebook and social media posts. You're happy, with a beautiful family." She seemed shocked and more than a little confused that I could be feeling anything like what she was going through and still appear calm and composed.

"Well, it's the truth. I do have a beautiful family and I like my job. But I think I've had these feelings of dread and doom for a while. Twenty-twenty was a tipping point, and I felt like it was time for a change ... and I had to do something."

"Wow. I'm shocked. But grateful you shared with me."

"Honestly, what you're feeling right now is okay. And you know it's okay to do something about it. You have two young children, and they come first. Look at the story of Dr. Breen, and her tragic end. We cannot let that happen to us. We have to protect each other."

"I know you're right, and I know there's an issue. I'm just scared to admit it, and I don't want to start medication."

I chuckled a bit, then explained, "I felt the same way and fought it for a while. I'm not saying you need to start medication but be open to talking to someone, perhaps a therapist or a counselor. Your job won't be in jeopardy, I promise. Do you have a PCP?"

"I do, but only go once per year ... barely."

I wasn't surprised. I told her, "We don't take good enough care of ourselves. We have to set the right example." She had tears. I continued. "Do you really think we are the only ones feeling this? Look at Dr. N, who has been here for almost thirty years. He looks miserable, disheveled, and just burned out. Do we really want to be like that? He's so cranky, and I'm convinced there is some depression or mood disorder."

"What made you want to change?"

I openly admitted that I didn't want to "risk being a bad husband or father and really needed to get it together."

"Is it helping?"

"Am I perfect? No. But am I better than I used to be? Definitely!"

We laughed and joked a bit more, and I shared with her some resources for local confidential workplace counselors. We hugged and promised to check in with each other. I later learned she had started seeing a therapist and was beginning to feel better. Progress continues.

The stories don't end there. When I look around in our profession, I see tenured physicians saying to me and others, "Go home and be with your kids. I lost those years and will never get them back. This field will suck it all out of you." I've seen other colleagues wind up divorced, separated, going through substance abuse and worse. Most important is that we respect one another's privacy. I do hope for the day when fear of social stigma no longer prevents physicians and health workers from speaking about and facing their struggles—and in so doing, showing others in our profession they can still be good doctors. At present, we are fortunate to have a movement organized around this effort, such as the Lorna Breen Foundation.

My friend and late colleague Dr. Jimmie Dancer always used to tell me, "Desai, you're married to another doctor. Go home and take care of her and your babies. This place is tough and will always be here. If you don't take care of that, you're going to lose it all—trust me."

I would listen and invariably reply, "You're right, Jimmie. I can't make everyone happy here."

"Ha! You never will."

During particularly demanding and exhausting shifts in the midst of those horrific COVID surges, he would send me texts and emails with inspirational quotes or Bible passages to motivate and ground me. They always came at just the right time, when I was most stressed or feeling most down. He seemed to have a sixth sense of what was going on. We didn't share the same faith, but the faith we shared was strong. He was wise and ahead of his time. I didn't always give him credit for what he had been through and seen with patients and colleagues, but he was the one who had seen it all. I wish I could go back and tell him how much we love and appreciate him. Jimmie also picked up on other clues, especially as they related to burnout among physicians. He would drag the younger doctors out of the office and demand that they come to the physician lounge with him "to get lunch"—as he knew that, like me, they too would not stop unless so advised by a trusted veteran physician. He truly was prescient in this regard, impressing upon us the importance of self-care, in particular our mental health and what can happen if we push ourselves too hard.

Now, I understand only too well. My eyes have been opened. Those in our field who struggle with burnout and issues affecting their mental health are at risk if they don't take remedial action. Ignoring the problem is dangerous. As someone who has gone through it, I want to lead by example. None of us is perfect, nor should we be expected to be, most particularly in our own eyes—no matter how high we insist on setting that bar. I say this even and especially as a doctor.

Chapter Six

Skin Color

Living with vitiligo is not easy to talk about, yet I'm sharing this important part of my life, as I realized during the events of 2020 how it has affected me and opened my eyes to the persistent issue of race. To be clear, I'm in no way embarrassed or ashamed by my skin color. It is a result of a disease process that affects a part of my body that people may see when they look at me. I never wanted to make it a bigger deal than it was, and it was ingrained in me by my family to not obsess about it. Vitiligo is an autoimmune disorder which attacks the melanocytes (the cells that produce melanin or pigment) in my body. So, over time, as the melanin-producing cells got destroyed, my skin developed white patches at varying stages. Today, my skin is essentially more than 90 percent depigmented.

I would be lying if I said I was not self-conscious or didn't have my guard up when someone does a double take as soon as they realize that my skin looks different. Why wouldn't I react that way? Aren't people conscious about their weight, scars, blemishes and other aspects of physical appearance?

To my benefit, I was sheltered, protected and shielded by my parents and also my brother, who simply never let anyone say anything around me about it while I was growing up. It was a blessing.

"Is anyone asking about your spots at school?" My father would check in regularly with me, referring to my patchy hypopigmented skin. Over time, the question became so routine, I'd barely notice. My mom never scolded him for asking, as she too wanted to know how things were going at school and to be sure that I was not being harassed. I would casually reply with a "no" or "nah" and move on, as this was the simple truth. I never was teased or ostracized for looking different because my skin was two colors. From my preteens to late adolescence, my vitiligo existed as localized patchy areas on my skin, specifically on my fingers, elbows, eyelids and knees. My school friends never asked me about it.

Sometimes a kid would notice in PE class, when I was wearing shorts, then ask, "Man, what happened to your knees?"

"It's sunburn scars," I would say.

"Crap! That looks like it would hurt!" would be the typical shocked reply, and then I'd shrug, ready to move on. That would be the end of it.

Looking back, if anyone did specifically ask about my skin, it never bothered me. I had coached myself, probably thanks to my family, that a shrug was to be the standard response: it says to the questioner, "I give it no mind." Ingrained in me early on was that having two different skin colors is no big deal and cannot define me, which I truly believed. Being a parent now, I can see that my parents were ahead of the curve in raising and coaching me to not feel different. It's beautiful. I like to think I would do the same for my children if they had anything similar or anything that might set them apart from the others. Frankly, I worry that if something ever were to happen, I would instantly become overprotective—and thereby risk making them self-conscious. My parents did the opposite, instilling in me a sense of normalcy at a time before easily accessible online blogs and support groups.

In the eighties and nineties, when I was growing up, having two different skin colors wasn't much of a topic. I lived in a relatively Caucasian community but went to public schools that were diverse with a large number of minority students. We were all together every day, as kids are at school, and I liked interacting with everyone. I never knew what it felt like to be treated differently because of skin color, and I never thought much about it at the time. Today, we talk about race, skin color, sex, and all the traits that distinguish us from one another as points of pride, as differences to be sharply defined. The idea that we all might be unified as one would doubtless sound strange to a child with vitiligo growing up today.

As a first-generation American in an Indian family, I became aware that my parents were also evading and proactively fighting a traditionally notorious social stigma. Vitiligo often is seen as taboo in the culture; many who have it are ostracized from their families, and some may be prevented from being married for fear that genetics plays a role and that vitiligo may be passed to future offspring. Aesthetically, too, in India it is seen as a major strike against the person. Societal taboos are powerful and not easily broken. Well aware of this, my parents nevertheless were determined to prevent me from falling into any of those traps. I would not be stigmatized. In this, they succeeded.

* * *

I remember, at age nine, in February 1993, seeing the Oprah Winfrey live interview with Michael Jackson, where he sat and talked candidly about his vitiligo. His recently changed appearance—and most importantly, his skin tone, which was considerably light—caused rumors to the effect that he'd been bleaching his skin, and here was an opportunity for him to address it in front of a worldwide audience of 90 million. As he began to explain, my mother gasped, which caught my attention: I saw in her relief mixed with shock, almost as if she were relieved to hear that someone as famous as Michael Jackson also struggled with this poorly understood condition. For Michael himself, it never seemed to be a focus, and I remember thinking about him and his vitiligo when the subject of his skin came up in conversation. I would hear people say, "He just wants to be White"—at which point I would always defend him. I knew perfectly well why, for instance, he needed an umbrella to protect himself from the sun's burning rays on those infamous days when he had to appear in court. The sun feels toxic on depigmented skin. Even a few minutes under a blazing sun will make those white patches turn instantly pink and then red, indicating a painful sunburn that may last for days. I can always feel the burning the moment I hit the sun. Sunscreen helps, but it's a constant battle to protect skin without melanin from UV rays. Blocking helps avoid the burning. Unlike other areas of pigmented skin, these patches cannot tan or bronze.

Since that famous interview, others have come out to discuss their vitiligo on social media and related platforms to a broad and support-ive audience, and I always feel validated when hearing about them. No one need ever struggle alone. It helps to connect. I didn't have that growing up, and while I never really felt the urge to discuss it, I like that this and similar topics can be shared in such forums. Not only does it take the focus off of you, but you can actively help someone else who may be struggling. To know what others are going through allows you to be part of a community.

With the murder of George Floyd and the emergence of racism as a twin pandemic in 2020, I decided I was ready to share my story. To be clear, I don't know what it feels like to be a Black man in America, judged and treated with bias solely on the basis of my race and color, but I do know what it feels like to be judged and seen differently based on color and appearance. Skin is the first thing we see in our inter-actions with one another, and that triggers immediate thoughts and reactions. For many, such responses include prejudgments. Unfair? Most likely. Unprecedented? Probably not. A simple look or a glance can be damning. Intentional or not, they are impossible to take back. A small exchange or interaction may be freighted with expectation that can all too easily lead to misunderstanding. While perhaps not the same as pure racism, judgment and bias are certainly at work.

* * *

In medical school, by the time I was in my late twenties, my vit-iligo began to explode. Busy and stressed with academics, I simply pushed my depigmenting skin into the background and tried to not let it distract me. It was beyond my control, something happening inside my body that made it seem as though my skin color was chang-ing before my eyes, in slow motion.

During the latter two years of medical school, I was around astute clinicians while I completed my clinical rotations in different special-ties. It was natural for them to notice, and some would diagnose my condition simply by looking at me and asking about it. While they cer-tainly weren't ignorant about disease and the disease process, many assumed that I didn't know what was going on with my body. What

I certainly *didn't* know—as no one ever can—is what was going on in their minds as they looked at me. This truth was brought home in stunning fashion one particular afternoon that I will never forget.

I was a third-year medical student then, on my family medicine rotation in Queens, New York. That afternoon, on a cold winter day in a busy outpatient primary care clinic, I was precepting patients with a few different attendings (that is, seeing a patient, getting a history, performing a physical exam, and coming up with a proposed plan, as a learner). The attending physician's task was to scrutinize my plan, give me feedback, and formally see the patient with me to finalize the treatment plan. As well can be imagined, my stress level was high; as a medical student, there was much I didn't know. Each situation was new, and the physicians with whom I worked had stark and often rigid personalities (making them harder to get along with). That's how it was, and we all had to get through it. Just being a medical student in itself is to be vulnerable.

"Mr. Desai, hang on right there!" shouted one of the attendings, someone who was known to be brash, curt and loud. I was in between patients and trying to help keep things moving.

"Okay, sure," I grudgingly replied, waiting with an aimless stare in the hallway. I assumed I was about to get reamed for a mistake or a clinical pearl I overlooked on a patient. I was nervous, my heart was racing, but I maintained my composure.

This attending, let's call him Dr. S, walked toward me. As he approached, he beckoned his female physician colleague and said, "Come with me. I need to show you something."

I knew his colleague from previous days, someone easy to talk to, sweet, even motherly. I always wanted to precept my patients with her, as she never became angry or frustrated. I felt safe with her. If he was bringing her, I reasoned, this couldn't be that bad.

The next forty-five seconds were the most humiliating, demoralizing and unacceptable that I'd experienced in all of my medical school training. Dr. S grabbed me by the arm and ordered, "Turn around." We were in the middle of the hallway with doctors, nurses and patients passing by.

Turning my neck and moving my shirt collar out of the way to get a better view of my skin, he said to his colleague, "Look at these patches on his skin. It looks like vitiligo."

Time collapsed in slow motion, as in a car crash. There I stood, in the middle of hallway traffic, being manipulated, as though I was a specimen in a lab, without my consent, without permission to be examined, let alone touched.

"Oh yes," she murmured. "Look at that."

I turned around instantly and told them, "Yes, I have vitiligo" in a voice cracked with embarrassment and anger.

Dr. S responded, "Yes, we can see that. It's obvious."

I felt my blood boil. My face was flushed, my heart pounding. I didn't know what to do. Here was this jackass, essentially patting himself on the back to impress a colleague, as if to say, *Here's something you don't see every day!* And the fact that I was his medical student somehow gave him this right—to stop me in my tracks, without my permission, and share me like some test subject, and in a hallway, no less!

I was mortified, and even worse, I was trapped. This was a hierarchy, and I had no power. He was the attending and I was the student. No one else was there to look after me, not really; the other attending, the one I thought motherly, just stood and smiled. I looked at her in horror, as if to say, *Save me, please!* with eyes that were fighting back tears.

"We doctors. Always looking at people through eyes of diagnosis. It's just what we do," was all she could say. She smiled at us both and rapidly walked away.

That was in the mid–2000s, and I can't imagine that such behavior would be tolerated today. That it was tolerated at all is partly the result of my having said nothing. I didn't stand up for myself; I didn't know how. Owing to certain nuances of the health system at that particular time and place, I chose to avoid what would have been a public confrontation. I was vulnerable as a medical student, worried about my evaluation, and needed to move forward without drama. That evening, walking alone to the subway station, I felt defeated. When I arrived home, I called a friend to vent, to let it out. I needed a sympathetic ear. My friend suggested I officially complain, stand up and say something. I said nothing. I felt powerless and hurt at the time.

*   *   *

Fast-forward a few years later, when I was working my intern year in residency in Dayton, Ohio, in the pediatric emergency room. Having gained experience and confidence, I still felt vulnerable and insecure in certain areas, with the added responsibility of being a new doctor. At this phase in our training, evaluations are conducted by an attending (that is, supervising) physician as part of the learning process. After each shift, we give the supervising doctor an evaluation sheet to fill out. The evaluations are helpful, and these physicians are well-trained to give constructive feedback. I certainly didn't mind it, and by then I had established a good rapport with most of the attendings. I was feeling comfortable and safe.

The forms used for evaluations are typically on green-colored paper. For some reason, the three-ring binder that held my evaluation forms contained a mix of green and white sheets. I didn't think anything of it, and most of the attending physicians didn't think much of it either—until that one evening, after my shift, when one of them made a remark.

I remember it was at midnight when I approached the supervising physician with my evaluation form, which happened to be white.

"Dr. E, I'm wrapping up here. Can we go over my evaluation form for today?"

"Yes, sure," he replied, grabbing my form. He looked at it twice with a puzzled expression, then laughed and said, "Oh, yeah, you also have vitiligo of your evaluation forms." He went on chuckling as he filled it out, then signed the form and handed it back.

There it was, once again. I was startled, in horror. *What did he just say?* He actually compared a white piece of paper to the color of my skin. Not once had we ever discussed my vitiligo, nor had he ever before acknowledged it. Yes, we had developed a good workplace rapport, so perhaps he felt enough at ease to make what he thought was a joke; even so, it was entirely inappropriate.

He looked straight at me after that line, and I faked a smirk and let out a "Yeah ..." but I felt as if I'd been kicked in the gut. He offered me some feedback, which I don't even remember, too shocked to process much of anything.

I grabbed my form, stuffed it in the binder, and quickly headed out to my car. I could feel myself choking up. I was mentally and physically exhausted, not only from working long hours but also simply trying to survive, single and alone in Ohio. I didn't need a reminder that the stark differences in my skin color were constantly being looked at and scrutinized—and by supervising physicians with no sense of tact, a situation I found appalling. What universe was I in? What century? I started to question basic things. Is it ever appropriate to make this type of remark, and if so, what right did this particular person have to make it? If he feels perfectly OK saying this to my face, what is he saying behind my back—and how do the others react? These are the people with whom I work every day, side by side; are they, too, laughing, smirking, making jokes? The answer is, no one has that right, but in that moment I was powerless. At the time, I just had to get through and come to grips with a stunning tone-deafness in others that may or may not have been due to a lack of diversity in a culture where such matters are never discussed.

Having experienced this firsthand, I well understand that patients with vitiligo are keen to know when people are looking at them and noticing their skin. It's the double takes, facial expressions and quick stares that we pick up on. Sometimes it is the unconscious reactions that sting the most.

I was in my fourth year of medical school taking a standardized patient exam: at this point, each fourth-year student is required to see and examine a set number of "patients" (who are actors) and write them up. We are graded pass or fail, but a passing grade is needed to graduate and match into residency. The standardized patient exam was offered only in a few select places around the country, and I came home to Atlanta to do mine.

On one of these encounters, the "patient" presented with a sore throat. I asked the routine questions, then proceeded to the physical

exam. My exam would be focused on her oral cavity and neck, looking for enlarged lymph nodes (swollen glands). I washed my hands and
asked permission to do a physical exam. As I approached the patient,
she stared at my hands, and the moment she noticed the patchy white
spots I could plainly see that she was disgusted. Remember that she
was an actor, someone trained in using facial expressions to convey
explicit emotions. This was clearly the person reacting, not the actor,
and she was physically moving away from me when I approached to
touch her neck (which I explained I would do). The body language was
unmistakable. It screamed, *Stay they hell away from me, and keep your
hands off me!*

I asked, "Are you OK?"

She answered, "Yes, doctor, please proceed" in a way I assumed
she felt she needed to, in order to help me get through the encounter.
I tried to not be distracted by her initial revulsion and kept on with
the exam. I had no choice but to keep moving forward, but I remember that face and her reaction to this day. One could argue that I was
overanalyzing or perhaps finding something that wasn't there, but her
physical response was undoubtedly genuine, and I believe that when
you sense or perceive another person's reflexive emotion, trust your
instinct—it's real. If any of my colleagues feel even a morsel of discrimination or bias from a patient, I listen closely and validate. The
worst thing you can say to that person is, "Oh, you're overreacting;
that didn't happen. Nothing was meant by that!"

* * *

In the spring of 2022, I was working with a patient who was a
retired physician. She was ill, having recently contracted COVID, and
struggling with respiratory issues. Her daughter, also a physician, was
in the room with us, advocating for her mother and asking appropriate questions. I was nearing ten years into practice as an attending,
and these kinds of frank conversations—about severe clinical consequences, end-of-life care and how best to navigate the different phases
of illness—was nothing new to me. In fact, I thrived on it. These are
some of the most challenging moments for a patient and the family

members, and my position at such times is to communicate, lead, and help to manage their care as illness progresses.

In this case, working with a family of physicians, there were added layers of questions and concerns. Naturally, this took considerably more time as both mother and daughter knew so much clinically that their questions were boundless. The patient herself was very astute and intelligent, which I respected. I had developed a rapport with them over a few days.

On the second day, just before my leaving the room (I was masked and wearing goggles), the patient looked at me with a smile. "One more question for you!"

"Sure, what's that?"

"Dr. Desai, you're Indian. Why is your skin so white? Are you mixed?"

My eyes must have started out of their sockets (thankfully hidden by the goggles). I paused. Out of the corner of my eye, I could see her daughter's horrified expression, a look that cried out, *Oh my God, I can't believe Mom just said that!*

Keeping calm and professional, I simply replied, "It's white because I have vitiligo."

The patient-physician smiled, as if she already knew the answer, and said, "Oh, OK."

"Yeah," I said, "and is there anything else I can help with?" She shook her head.

Walking out of the room, I just rolled my eyes. This time I didn't feel powerless. In fact, I now felt empowered. In this instance, I could openly share what was going on with my skin, to answer this person's question. I didn't change the subject. My bluntness may have made the patient feel awkward, but the careless questioning made it that much more awkward and uncomfortable for me.

* * *

These are but a few examples of what I mean by intrinsic racism and what some of us have to deal with on the professional level. I share my experiences not for sympathy but rather to show how it's possible to go from powerless to powerful in society and the workplace. The events of 2020 marked a turning point. I am no longer afraid or too shy to discuss vitiligo and the difference it has created for me. What once had been a taboo topic no longer is taboo. People will say things. It's our nature. How we ask a question and choose our words is up to us, and this includes our responses. What others say to me is out of my control, but I certainly am not powerless in that situation. Whether or not I feel it right or appropriate, if and when I'm asked about my skin, I'm now at a place where I feel empowered to share the reality of what's going on. I can be simple and truthful. I can be direct. No, I'm not going to naturally bring it up, but the minute it does come up, I'm going to say something. I will explain the condition and stand up for myself.

I don't feel that patients treat me any differently when they become aware of my vitiligo, but the fact of it brings me to a deeper question: What do patients necessarily assume the moment they see us enter their rooms? If my skin were a shade of brown, would they assume I'm Indian and not ask the question? Or, if my skin tone was black, would they assume I'm African American? Would that then cause them to have a different expectation of me, and would my presence produce a different reaction? The answer to all of these questions may well be yes.

The events of 2020 certainly sparked a movement. In the midst of the COVID chaos and all that I was going through on the personal and professional front, I woke up to the reality that, while I make no claim to having suffered from overt racism, I can still be judged and scrutinized on the basis of my skin color. Some of these are microaggressions, others are more straightforward. Yet things are changing. People are more aware. We haven't "solved" the issues surrounding racism but we are slowly creating ways to avoid the worst excesses of discrimination and give people a voice and platform to halt its progress. When I compare my experiences with vitiligo to those whose lives have been damaged by out-and-out racism, they are not at all the same, yet they share one important aspect: that of being noticed for having different skin and the altered expectation of a person that goes along with that. It happens daily to anyone being so judged. Though I never suffered a career setback because my skin looks different, I cannot say the same for others. The good news is that within our current healthcare system and structure, there is a power to change and adapt. That will come with time.

*   *   *

On a professional level, I have never allowed my condition to define me. How, then, you might ask, has vitiligo affected my personal life? In Yogita, I have a loving and accepting partner, one who has neither judged me nor ever had biased feelings against me for my skin, and we share a physical and emotional attraction. I was upfront at the beginning of our relationship as to what was going on and she accepted me. To me, that is everything, and to this day, it's never been a barrier. When we were dating, I remember that additional areas of my skin were depigmenting. In a moment of frustration and self-doubt, I asked her, "What are you going to do ten years from now if my entire body is depigmented?"

"Well, you, me, and the kids will deal with it," is how she responded.

I think that was my way of testing the waters to make sure she knew what could happen. The reality is, it *has* happened: my skin is now more than 90 percent depigmented. We are together now as a family of four. Even in pictures today, I can clearly see the differences in my skin tone from that of my children. I try not to fixate on or think too much about it.

I do wonder what my children will think in the coming years. When will they begin to question or ask why my skin is different? And how do I prepare them? My younger one is only three, so he doesn't know any better. Kaiya is now seven, and she certainly is more aware. What she knows for sure is that Daddy has to be careful in the sun, as she frequently reminds me, "Daddy, did you wear sunscreen?" So far, she's never asked why.

As parents of two young children, Yogita and I speak with one voice when it comes to the need for them to grow up with tolerance and diversity. We are a minority as Indians, and we want Kaiya, and soon Kaveh, to know and accept people of all races and ethnicities. I find it true, as the saying goes, that kids don't see color; having a family has opened my eyes to this fact, that children are born to accept and be around others and that they are able, early on, to "play with everyone." It's beautiful to see, and we want those accepting, loving eyes and natures to continue throughout their lives. We will do whatever we can to foster those values in our children. Since racism is a behavior that is learned, it therefore must never be taught.

I'd had an ongoing dialogue with myself for years about how and when to tell Kaiya about my vitiligo in a way that she would understand. Yogita always urged that I not make it a big deal but that however I decided to handle it was up to me. In our family, we typically read to our kids before bed, and one evening I was presented with an opportunity.

We were reading a book that Kaiya checked out from the library about people around the world and all the differences among us. The theme was how all the differences make us one. As Kaiya and I together turned the page, I saw there illustrated a young lady whose skin is shaded two colors. Clearly, she has vitiligo. Yogita and I look at each other. Now, she seemed to suggest with a smile in her eyes, might be a good time to talk about it. I took a few calming breaths to prepare myself for what was to be a defining moment between me and my daughter. I was nervous.

As soon as we finished reading that page, I stopped Kaiya.

"Hey, honey, wait just a minute. I want to show you something on this page and talk about it."

"What, Daddy?!" She sounded slightly annoyed that I was holding up the reading.

"You see this girl here, and how her skin is two colors, black and white?"

"Umm, yeah," she said, pushing me to hurry.

"She has *vitiligo*, a skin condition, where your skin turns white. That's what Daddy has."

We all paused. I felt so free after saying that. Yogita was smiling a proud, beaming smile; I was emotional, primed and ready for questions.

Waiting for a response, I was all set for a longer conversation coming my way. This was the time I would always remember. Instead, Kaiya squinted her eyes, shrugged, and said, "Okay!" then she turned the page and asked that we keep on reading. What?! That was it? She didn't want to know anything more, or perhaps she didn't need to; moreover, she never asked about it again. Instead, she moved on to the following page and on with the story. I know she understood, but she didn't care enough to inquire any further. It made no difference in her eyes; I was Daddy. That simple.

Yogita and I just smiled at each other, as if to say, *Well, that was anticlimactic!* Kids are intuitive. I'm sure Kaiya knew that something was different long before this, but she never felt a need to question or make it a big deal. I haven't brought it up since then and may not need to again. I'm sure it will come up in conversation, but so far, my condition hasn't affected her in any significant way. It's clear that for Kaiya, vitiligo is not a defining characteristic, nor should it be. My dream is that this inherent acceptance continues as she interacts with more and more people.

* * *

I can see that my daughter, now in first grade, doesn't question or even especially notice another person's skin. If I were to ask her where a friend is from, if that friend has a non–American-sounding name, she has to stop and think about it. The world, though, sooner or later sets us apart, usually on the basis of color. As a colleague once said ruefully, "the world we live in is black and white."

The summer of 2020 was an epiphany for me, not just as a father and frontline physician during COVID but also as someone who fully came to recognize the systemic racism that had gone on around me my entire life. In those "advanced classes" that lacked minority students, were those students ever even given a chance? What about my fellow physicians who fall into that same category—are they, too, always included? I often think about the Black nurse getting yelled at and insulted by a prejudiced White patient—how is our system caring for her? And what about the Asian nurse who happened to have an accent, who spoke proficient English, getting reamed by a patient who claimed that she couldn't be understood? These manifold micro-aggressions and behaviors that separate and alienate us by race and ethnicity continue to plague us in healthcare and beyond. Yet, with awareness further raised by the climactic events of 2020, we are positioning ourselves to be more receptive to diversity without the usual bias. It doesn't happen overnight; the only requirement is willingness. While such awareness and acceptance may be slow in coming in healthcare due to constant chaos and competing priorities, change indeed is happening.

* * *

Having lived and grown up with vitiligo, I can safely say that, for the most part, I'm at acceptance. (As with any disease, it comes with surprises.) It continues to give me insight. While it's clear, for instance, that I am Indian and my skin should be brown, I don't speak with an accent, and the fact that vitiligo allows me at times to pass as Caucasian is often an advantage. That it confuses some people, who may wonder if I'm mixed with Indian and American blood, that too can be advantageous, as it can provide an opportunity for learning.

Until relatively recently, I'd always viewed having depigmenting skin as a disadvantage, and it does still present me with uncomfortable situations. Yet, the idea that my vitiligo is working against me simply isn't true, and experience proves it. Having depigmented skin may well have created an advantage that I never fully acknowledged until the past few years—one that has always been there. There's the idea of "White-passing" that may have created an advantage for me so I avoided any bias or preconceived notions from being "brown."

* * *

Looking back on my years in residency, I often wonder if I've benefited from institutionalized racism, in my case, vitiligo camouflaging my ethnicity. That I've gained an advantage from appearing White is an uncomfortable possibility. I have no control over what others assume when they see me and draw conclusions. Yet, the fact that some brown people may pass for White in our society is undeniable. Who knows if that happened with me? Was I receiving the benefits that accrue to those who blend in with this (then) largely White population, throughout my residency? It's entirely possible.

Bias from patients toward non–White physicians is nothing new, nor has it abated. In such patients, the moment color is perceived, their attitude and demeanor noticeably change. This is as true today as it was when I started out as a medical student. The doctors and nurses and medical staff, who are there to protect and care for every patient, deal daily with a range of discriminatory bias when they happen to have different-colored skin. I've heard colleagues' reports and witnessed this firsthand, and it's been eye-opening.

"Get out of here, I don't want someone like you in my room," is a common refrain when a hijab is spotted or the health provider entering is Black. We are trained in how to respond to such patients. We speak evenly and firmly, with a stolid expression.

"Okay," we say (in this case, a Muslim doctor), "I'm here to help you. Are you going to let me examine you and take care of you?"

"Do the minimum you need to and just leave!" comes the reply, usually issued as a hostile demand.

In this instance, my colleague did more than the minimum and made excellent clinical decisions that ultimately saved the patient's life, but it wasn't without damage to her morale and identity.

As this doctor and I decompressed, it was clear that institutional change is needed, particularly after the upheavals of 2020 and all that followed. The need for initiatives on equity and inclusion are more pressing than ever, especially in the workplace. I can't help but wonder, though, if advantages gained by racial passing, even unwittingly, continue to give certain individuals an edge, even as we champion diversity.

How much of this is still going on can be difficult to pinpoint in practice. A change, for instance, in a patient's demeanor may have nothing to do with skin tone. Then again, if it does, and the patient stays quiet, how would I or any of us even know? Take, for example, one of my patients, with whom I've established an excellent rapport:

I move on, and the doctor who takes over for me, who happens not to be White, has an entirely different patient experience, one that is hostile and negative. Taking into account variables such as bedside manner, communication style and related factors—none of which adequately explains the sudden shift in this patient's attitude—what am I left to conclude? Perception as it relates to expectation on the part of the patient must have played a role. My colleague and I—neither of us is White—are relatively equal in our approach and care style. Is racial passing helping me in subtle ways that can't be seen?

The reality is complex and not easy to fathom, much less talk about. Even harder to know is to what extent this has touched my life. The events of 2020 have been a catalyst for me to open my eyes to what is around me. As societal crises unfold and COVID surges rebound, I'm forced to confront inequities on all fronts. It isn't just skin. Male doctors, for instance, don't face the same challenges as female physicians, who often are not treated with the same dignity and respect. Countless times, my wife, Yogita, as a female doctor, has been mistaken for a nurse or tech. Economic inequities abound as well. The list goes on and on.

There isn't one solution to it all. Being open to dialogue is an important first step. Expressing concerns as they arise in the moment, listening and following through with concrete action are some of the ways that will help move us to a more equitable place. We certainly are in a better position for broader acceptance than we were ten years ago. Today, I have a clearer view, thanks in no small part to the last three years, in my daily interactions with and support of my colleagues. And from a patient care standpoint, I am ever more focused to ensure that my approach is equitable and that I advocate for all. I remain a work in progress. I see now what I had not seen before.

CHAPTER SEVEN

Divided

"Daddy, can I go back to school?" pleaded my four-year-old. "I miss my friends ... staying at home is boring. Not fair!" These were constant complaints during her tantrums and meltdowns. She wasn't alone. Millions of children around the country wanted to go back to school.

Yogita and I were able to find a preschool tutor for Kaiya and we partnered with the family of one of her friends, alternating half-days at one another's home for "minischool." The arrangement provided some much-needed structure in an environment that was verging on chaotic. We were all still adapting to life turned upside down. Kaveh, in the meantime, was a growing infant under strict new protocols. He never left the house except to be taken for brief walks in his stroller. He wasn't exposed to people or public places. He was an example of what was coming to be known as a "pandemic baby": isolated, shielded and homebound.

"Why aren't you sending your child back to school? COVID doesn't affect children!" is the mantra I would hear in fall 2020, when the new hybrid plans at the start of school had begun to be implemented. "This is so blown out of proportion," declared frustrated others. Coming to terms with such statements and attitudes was more and more difficult, if not impossible, for me. How could one convince such people otherwise? Trying to explain what was truly happening with regard to the pandemic and public health was becoming a fool's errand. I couldn't duck the conversation, either; these were now confrontations. Up against such willful ignorance, the likes of which I'd not seen before, I'd get overwhelmed—blood would rush through my body, muscles would tighten, and inside, I'd begin to rage.

The reality is that most people haven't witnessed the degree of suffering caused by COVID-19 in hospitalized patients. They haven't seen the extent of it firsthand: patients gasping for air, shaking and screaming, "I can't breathe!" They haven't witnessed families torn apart when their loved ones are hospitalized and intubated. This was certainly *not* blown out of proportion, but in this case, bizarrely, arguing facts was useless. It was a brain drain. In the teeth of all this—what was now becoming "controversial"—Yogita and I had to refocus our energies on what was right for our own family and loved ones.

* * *

The pandemic brought unprecedented changes for so many. It affected careers. Yogita had been transitioning into a new position before the pandemic and all its restrictions, and now, in fall 2020, she needed to travel. She was leaving the academic group and joining a private practice where she would focus on the management and treatment of pelvic pain, which had developed into her clinical niche and passion. This was yet another major life change for our family, but she'd worked hard for this and the time was right. We all were happy and supportive. It was a step up as well as a position with better hours that allowed her to be home at a regular time on evenings and weekends. The problem was, she was expected to go to Miami for training in the midst of the second surge.

"I want you and the kids to come with me when I go to Miami for my training. Kaveh needs me. I'm still nursing. I can't leave the kids for a week." This was the opening of what would become a weeks-long conversation between us. She was feeling tremendous guilt at the prospect of leaving her nursing six-month-old, and she wanted her family with her for the trip, but I was not sold on the idea of traveling. Frankly, I was against it. Florida in general and Miami in particular had become a hotspot by late summer–early fall 2020. How could we be safe there with two small kids? Are we to drive eleven hours with screaming children in the car or fly and expose them to COVID? Once arrived, what do we do with them? Do we remain confined in the hotel room while Yogita is off at training all day? Each anxious question generated a new one, for which there appeared to be no easy answer. While all this was going through my mind, I struggled with how much I should share with Yogita, whose desire that we join her came straight from the heart. To me, though, traveling as a family seemed unwise.

I had already cleared my calendar for that week. The timing was impeccable, as I desperately needed a break from work. What I hadn't factored in was travel and especially not to a COVID hotspot with family. After much deep discussion and many tears, we arrived at a decision: I would stay behind with the kids and Yogita would go to Miami by herself.

I was relieved, for two reasons: we were given a reprieve from the stress involved with travel, and we would not be exposing ourselves. I was tired. I wanted to stay at home, sleep in my bed, do daily routines with the kids. Fear of my young ones getting COVID, especially our six-month-old, haunted me day and night. While it was true no significant surge of pediatric hospitalizations due to COVID appeared at this point, even one hospitalization or severe illness in a child presented too much risk for me. I felt guilty enough at the prospect of exposing them to anything I may have brought home from work.

Dressed in clean scrubs, N95 mask, eye shield and gloves, Yogita flew to Miami. Kaiya understood that Mommy was going away for one week and that she and her brother would be home with Daddy. Looking into tear-filled eyes, I told Yogita how much we loved her and how proud we were, reassuring her that all would be well on the home front. She wasn't worried, she said, but heartbroken to be leaving us, especially now.

That whole week, we FaceTimed every day and talked and texted constantly. It was good for me in so many ways: I could work on more one-on-one sleep training for Kaveh and get into the groove of my children's routines. It was so gratifying, just being a dad for that week. I was able to bond with them in a way I hadn't done since the pandemic began. I learned new things about Kaveh's daily life, aspects of which I'd been ignorant of up to now. It truly felt as if sunshine had broken into a room that had too long been dark.

* * *

By the middle of fall 2020, the second surge had passed, with cases trending downward. A degree of routine had established itself with COVID. At the hospital and across the nation, we had become better with treatments and developing remedial agents to help combat the original virus. But it was *not* over. We all understood there was no way out of this until we had a vaccine. Or so we thought.

The country was on edge. New safety protocols suggested by the CDC and others were being challenged by people who demanded that their lives return to normal. Imperfect understanding created the perfect storm, which was quickly exploited by self-interested groups or those who might profit from the chaos. Disunity, in this case, offered a political advantage, and misinformation about the disease had begun to divide people into separate camps. Battlegrounds began to form around public health issues, such as masking mandates and the opening of schools. Countless districts came up with hybrid plans that continued to be challenged in divided communities. Parents scrambled to arrange for childcare and improvised alternative options. Working from home had become the new normal. Chaos loomed in a world that strived to go back to life before COVID.

We weren't ready to go back. Though schools needed to reopen, questions remained about safety. True, there had been a generalized decrease and plateauing of COVID numbers and to some degree people started to relax, but my world was marked by increasing fear. We still hadn't developed a vaccine, yet mitigation practices were quickly dropping off in communities as the holidays neared. Predictor models, ever at risk of being inaccurate or flawed, nevertheless foretold a significant COVID surge with increased hospitalizations in the winter months. One such model predicted a 20 percent increase in hospitalizations in my area from the previous summer surge.

With such dire forecasts in mind, it was all I could do not to panic. As leader of my group, I needed to prepare. Not only were we having staffing issues, but I was also now questioning how we would sustain if those predictions turned out to be accurate. We were already seeing higher volumes of patients, some of whom had not seen a healthcare provider in more than a year who were lost to follow-up or had not sought medical care due to changes, fears and reluctance involving the pandemic. These patients had complex medical needs, and our health-care teams were in constant demand. How could we split our time, efforts, focus and resources to handle both this baseline hospital population with what could be a tsunami of new COVID patients? Something would have to give.

We were preparing for disaster. Hospitals formed groups and committees to work through supply chain issues, as well as to ensure staffing needs were met (e.g., through redeployments) and to requisition PPE—anticipating likely shortages. It felt like preparing for a category 5 hurricane, but rather than hitting us all at once, this storm would surge and continue for weeks, intensifying in ferocity as it picked up speed. Adding to our woes was the dreaded expectation that with COVID, we were in it for the long haul. During that fall, the way in which the virus was spreading left us breathless, with no time to regroup. The storm just kept hitting us.

Countless hours were spent in meetings, planning staffing contingencies for my group. Each creative scenario carried pitfalls. There was no magic solution, no way to run a smooth operation. Where one staffing plan might lead to gaps in real time, another left our workers without any breaks, no relief in a high-volume flood of patients. I felt I was simply restacking the cards in a house that could fall at any minute.

Another unrelieved point of stress was a constant fear that multiple physicians might get sick with COVID all at once. If so, that would destroy our operations. No pool of substitute doctors is out there ready to step in, and we at the hospital cannot work safely for days on end filling in for one another. The hospitalist model was developed and premised on the idea of time off to rest from the stress brought about by intensive hospital work. How could we possibly sustain in the event that our workforce became rapidly depleted due to illness? Would we be expected to see twenty-five to thirty patients at once, in a hospital setting? If so, that would be asking the impossible, and I felt that permanent weight on my shoulders.

* * *

"I can't do this anymore. I've found another position where I can work from home," announced an exhausted colleague in November 2020.

"Wow," I muttered, eyes wide with the news, thinking, *How am I going to fill this staffing gap?*

"They need me to start in two weeks, and I don't think that I can work the holidays this year as we scheduled. Dhaval.... I'm tired and have been practicing hospital medicine so many years. It's never been like this. I need something new."

"I understand. I get it. This is tough, and you must focus on you," I replied, acknowledging her reality but at the same time dreading what that implied. If she had already reached this point, how might that impact the others? Would they too seek a career change soon? We knew what was coming and were desperately short of staff; filling shifts had become a daily challenge. Now I had to worry about attrition.

"Hospital life is too different. Why should I stay and work in an area where I'm constantly exposing myself to this virus and take it home to my loved ones, who are immunocompromised? This job is not my life. My life is at home. I'm just done!" she exclaimed.

I listened, intent. The doctor wasn't finished.

"And know that I'm worried about you. You give way too much here. You look exhausted, and you have *another* family, at home. This place will break you," she warned. "You better watch it."

I knew she's right. I hadn't yet pivoted. I continued to give more than was good for my health, both mental and physical. How could I not, though, under the present circumstance? This was the unremitting, difficult question, in spite of the work I'd done facing just that, in the past year, dealing with all the stress. I knew in my bones I would never walk away, yet I also knew that what she was telling me was true: I had to find a better balance. Survival depends on it.

Another related disturbing development in our hospital community was the sudden early retirement of nurses and respiratory therapists, who were leaving in droves for nonhospital opportunities. *It's just not worth it to me* and *My family matters more* were constant refrains. With such high turnover and unfamiliar travel nurses and staff coming in, it became nearly impossible to build trust. Onboarding a medical team takes time, as does establishing rapport and good relationships. Under these unusual conditions, staff that had been working on the front line for years were suddenly faced with brand-new hires earning far more pay. It was demoralizing for them and demoralizing to see. Travel gigs are absurdly lucrative, so much so that I often wonder if a doctor could work as a travel nurse during time off to make even greater heaps of cash (plus travel expenses) with less medical legal risk. It was wild. The result of this topsy-turvy situation was to incentivize leaving the local hospital workforce, as so many did, not just here, but all over the country.

*   *   *

Doomscrolling was now a favorite pastime, and it often accompanied disaster planning. Indeed, the two went hand in hand. My Twitter feeds were filled with anecdotes about COVID cases and hospitals that were struggling to maintain staff. I wouldn't go as far as to call it schadenfreude, but I felt weirdly comforted knowing we weren't the only ones battling these and similar issues. Incessantly checking social media to read up on others' disasters in real time was disturbing, however, and my colleagues noticed. Many strongly suggested that I get off social media, that it was making me too anxious. For me, it wasn't so much seeing those worst-case scenarios happen as it was experiencing a camaraderie with my fellow doctors, who were just as stymied, just as perplexed. I needed to be connected, to know they were there, even though—and maybe even because—they were strangers. Disturbing, as I said, but also necessary. My silver lining in the midst of this duress is that we physicians were going through it together.

While attrition was high, not everybody left. Those frontline workers who elected to stay did so at no small cost. Countless conversations were devoted to fatigue and fear of taking COVID home. There is no getting used to it. Fatigue is fatigue, and it wears you out, under any circumstance. Fear exacerbates what is already stressed, not only in individuals but also in groups—and in my case, my team. As leader, I was responsible for managing such pressures, and in fall 2020, they were severe. At that time, we started our fiscal year, which typically involves a renewal of energy, focus and priorities. The previous seven months had been consumed by the pandemic, with our primary focus on trying to survive.

Now, I needed to reorder those priorities, at the same time managing the pandemic for our group. There was a push for team leaders to create a sense of normalcy under panic conditions—above all, to help mitigate the deleterious effects of anxiety and fear among hospital workers but also to create and implement new strategies and initiatives. From my perspective—the front line of COVID, with an expected and near certain winter surge—it was hard to fathom adding more to our plates at a time when we were already going above and beyond.

We were still without a vaccine. Patients were dying in ever greater numbers. I was still in survival mode and neither motivated nor interested to plan new projects and initiatives. Some days, I could barely function. I argued to my higher-ups that new projects and increased expectations only puts more pressure on an already stressed physician or nurse. The counterargument is that a new initiative perhaps could shift one's mind away from COVID and in that way renew interest in one's career and opportunities. Maybe it would work for some. I had my doubts.

I admired those who could look beyond the pandemic and coached myself to lead like them by motivating my group to focus on themselves with strategies to build their careers. Accordingly, I opened the new fiscal year with a primary focus on navigating the pandemic while working on creative strategic initiatives to make us as productive a group as possible. While it felt good, setting this new tone, I remained cautious about shifting focus away from COVID—at the same time trying as much as I could to instill a sense of hope. I often counsel patients to remain cautiously optimistic when facing a grim prognosis, offering them a degree of hope while trying to accept and acknowledge reality. That cautious approach proved correct when the surge hit us in December 2020 and everything once more spiraled into chaos.

* * *

As communities grappled and became increasingly divided over the extent and severity of the new coronavirus, the national response had yet to be coordinated. The CDC had offered guidelines about the importance of masking and social distancing and the necessity of frequent, thorough hand-washing, but implementation proved difficult. People tend to argue when you tell them what to do, never mind if the purpose is to mitigate risk. That the virus was lethal was being argued as well, some even calling it a hoax. Even so, the nation was attempting to adapt its infrastructure to survive in the midst of this outbreak. Much of that involved a new set of protocols with which communities and individuals were expected to comply. In so doing, we protect not just ourselves but one another, and in this way, help to guard against transmitting disease. Compliance, therefore, was a shared responsibility, and in those days, before we had a vaccine, it meant survival. This was life or death.

Yet, despite the chaotic atmosphere and daily tragedies we'd experienced at the hospital throughout the first half of 2020, disbelief and doubt over COVID-19 continued to be sown at the national level and in communities. Once it became clear that political interests could be served by underplaying COVID's most serious risks, the messaging started to change at the senior-most levels of the administration about public health protocols. Masking and isolation guidelines were now in dispute and—alarmingly for us—subject to change, depending on the prevailing views and notions of various state and federal officials. The public was confused. Trusted agencies such as the CDC were suddenly being brought into question, and their lack of coordinated messaging didn't help. Bear in mind that as doctors, we didn't yet fully know COVID, but what we did know about how to mitigate transmission was now being actively undermined by officials advantaged by the spread of misinformation. Cable news and social media, reporting from all sides, disseminated their views into vast niche markets where everything is subject to suspicion and doubt—places where truth is often up for grabs. In these ways, at that time, trust in the scientific and medical community, along with expertise itself, began to dissipate. So much had changed in such a short amount of time.

One Sunday morning that fall, while masked and shopping at the local grocery store, I noticed the store clerk posted at the entrance reminding every person coming in to wear a mask. A couple in their fifties walked past without masks and were politely asked to put them on. The employee had extra masks and was offering them to the couple, if needed.

"Ugh. Not necessary—and I should have a choice!" exclaimed the husband.

"Just put it on and let's get in and out. This is ridiculous," the wife tried to calm him.

Overhearing these remarks, I rolled my eyes then winked at the store clerk and thanked him for being there. A few minutes later, I spotted that same couple chatting in the aisle with their masks pulled down to their necks. I walked by them, glared, and again rolled my eyes. They didn't see or hear me but as I quickly moved past, I muttered out loud, "Well, there are my next two patients!"

To this day, it still angers me. Throughout the community, I would encounter this mindset, this attitude of stubborn resistance to help protect oneself and others from contracting a virus known to send people into hospitals and their graves. It was maddening to see the public safety messaging so willfully ignored. More and more, I'd see people out and about without a mask, mingling and socializing in crowded public places, and then, too, I'd be stared at and judged for wearing a mask—as if I were the problem, infringing on their rights. Public health be damned. This was now about an individual's right to choose, and masking mandates were deemed government overreach. Cries of *Liberty!* were being invoked, stoked by reckless media folks and feckless politicians.

Who knew that masking and soon-to-come vaccines could so divide us? Yet here we are. You might think that by now, having seen the numbers of COVID-related deaths and long-term suffering for which there is still no cure, that people would be less entrenched in their view that the pandemic is a hoax and that COVID is no different from the common cold. *No different from the flu* is the typical view, and it persists. Those who subscribe to such beliefs—and they are legion—would come to the hospital and refuse to wear masks; some even called it a conspiracy. Families of hospitalized patients would be outraged when told that they couldn't enter without a mask and frequently became irate and abusive. One family member stormed out of the building, screaming at the top of her lungs, "You will NOT TAKE AWAY MY FREEDOM with these STUPID MASKS!" We too were frustrated, but for different reasons: those we were trying to help were taking it out on us.

One patient went so far as to argue, "Look, I know you get more money if you keep me in the hospital with COVID for another day. Just let me go home."

His accusation left me momentarily speechless.

"Sir," I began, "nothing could be further from the truth. I have nothing to do with compensation and reimbursement—and I assure you that I want you home as soon as possible!" From the look on his face, he remained unconvinced.

I saw at once what was happening. In ever greater numbers, people who were showing up at the hospital with COVID had been told they were not really sick. Once they arrived, we were being accused of monetizing their illness. It was all a grand conspiracy and we were part of it, coordinating with government agencies to maximize profit. They, of course, were the victims. Others insisted that our funding increased with each COVID-related death—a morbid incentive. Such beliefs are impossible to counter with sane argument; logic and reason are of no use. Additional frustrations involved our getting berated for not getting back to families soon enough with updates. We didn't lack for compassion, but the wall of anger against us was staggering. Any attempts to disabuse such folks of their dark beliefs only made things worse for everyone. I wondered how my colleagues up north were faring, if they had encountered such profound mistrust.

Incredibly, we were beginning to see *hospitalized* COVID patients argue with clinicians about which treatments they would and would not be willing to receive. Not only was our expertise in doubt, but we were also now being told by certain COVID patients how to treat them. While many people certainly did trust us—those who would gasp for air, desperately weak, and plead for anything to make them feel better—there were also those who resisted. In such cases, they would try to pick and choose what treatment they wanted administered.

I've always been an advocate for patient-centered care and shared decision-making, but, to this day, I struggle with those who choose to refuse recommended treatment for COVID. At one point, a patient in his eighties who was otherwise healthy was admitted to our hospital for COVID. On his explicit instructions, his family were his medical proxies and we were obliged to follow their decisions regarding treatments and other aspects of his care. In this case, his family were the ones refusing remdesivir and other recommended treatments for him.

"Doctor, we respect you, but we have read extensively about remdesivir, and he's just not getting it," concluded the daughter of this elder patient, making clear there would be no further discussion with regard to that specific medication. On day seven of his illness, he had the classic cytokine storm—a condition that develops when the immune system responds too aggressively to infection—and rapidly decompensated and died. I remain convinced that had this patient been given remdesivir or one of the monoclonal antibody treatments as he started to qualify with increasing disease severity, he would have had a much greater chance at surviving.

Patients instead would demand ivermectin—a drug commonly used to treat parasitic infections—asking for "evidence" that it does *not* work rather than to follow any other treatment. Our clinical judgment, based on what we were seeing in the progression of COVID not just in our population but nationwide, thus was disregarded by such patients and their families who refused to comply with any treatment plan other than what they themselves suggested.

People sometimes make the counterargument that a COVID patient who refuses treatment is no different than any other noncompliant patient, such as the diabetic who doesn't take insulin, for instance, or the patient suffering with congestive heart failure who drinks too much fluid or has too much salt. From the point of view of hospital admission, the difference is profound. In the latter two examples, one simply accepts the insulin and diuretics, respectively, upon arrival. The COVID patients who refuse treatment, however, are at the sickest phase of the disease, where the medicines and treatments they refuse could help them. They're locked in a state of disbelief at a critical moment in their care. To run up against this impenetrable wall left me feeling defeated and helpless.

Noncompliance and resistance to a hospital's masking policy affects everyone, inside and outside the hospital, regardless of a person's health at point of entry. This basic fact about transmissibility of infectious disease was getting lost in the "controversy" over so-called mandates—a word that had come to mean infringement on one's rights. Through lack of trust, in both authority and the principles of science, many simply refused to believe what was being told to them. They felt, even righteously so, that in their case, hospital policy didn't apply. This included those being admitted for non–COVID reasons, many of whom didn't or wouldn't understand. After all, went their reasoning, they didn't have COVID. They were in the hospital for something else. Why wear a mask? Explanations seemed only to anger such patients and accompanying visitors, who were dismissive and frustrated that I was speaking to them through an N95 mask.

These and related types of arguments with clinicians and hospital staff weren't limited to any single demographic or age group. Rather, we were seeing it across the board. Clearly, there can be no pleasing everyone, but this was different. It wasn't a matter of winning someone over, no longer about that difficult phone call to family or whether or not a patient was being treated for COVID. While cooperation and empathy with our workers continued, public anger was mounting. Things had reached the point where one sour interaction could ruin hours of work, making us all feel demoralized. Not only were we fighting a pandemic and disease, but now we were fighting people—and they were many—who could not accept the gravity of the situation and the well-known lethal and long-term unknown consequences with which we all were dealing. None of this was going to be short-lived until everyone bought into a comprehensive strategy to mitigate against this novel, now mutating, virus.

* * *

At the start of the pandemic, my healthcare colleagues and I were being hailed as heroes but now the tone had softened and was disappearing rapidly. Those first few months, tough as they were on so many levels, were notable for the degree and intensity of people's gratitude, not only from the individuals we helped, but also from a community that was rallying and advocating for healthcare workers. Bells were ringing nightly for those on the front line in New York City at an appointed hour, when people would open their windows to cheer us on—and we heard them all the way in Atlanta. Here, too, were celebrations and donations for healthcare workers with food and necessities. Signs across the city beamed thanks for everyone working on the COVID front line. We felt it, and those feelings mattered; community spirit gave us purpose and strength in a time and place where we needed it most.

That was then. As COVID continues to plague society, that idea of community—that we are going through this together—has been muddled, if not entirely lost. Our worlds inside hospitals, clinics and medical facilities have been fundamentally altered in ways that negatively affect our practice. By fall 2020, what used to be a safe assumption about treatment plans and patient care was no longer in play and the landscape so changed that we were losing experienced workers at an unsustainable rate. The building blocks of a healthcare system are its workers and the talent they bring. Theirs is a unique set of skills, honed over years in the field of medicine to heal and care for a patient. These keystones of our practice had never before been so challenged and jeopardized, and the subsequent fallout, the result of unceasing assaults on our system, has been devastating. The loss of experienced workers of twenty to thirty years simply cannot be replaced. Bringing in a junior workforce means less experienced people in positions that take years in which to develop proficiency. Such moves rarely come without costs.

Healthcare is a fundamental need in a community, and unless we have stable access to it, we can neither live in nor have a healthy society. Responsibility and action at the community level to focus on and maintain public health includes following healthcare guidance such as masking, timely vaccinations and listening to experts. Trust is a must. Without most of the community on board, aligning to prevent the spread of COVID-19 and its manifold variant strains, it persists and will continue to disrupt us.

The writing on the hospital wall is clear. Staffing has forever changed, leading to care that is less than optimal until the talent pool is increased. The present situation will continue to erode as long as financial incentives exist to draw our best-skilled and most experienced workers away and into other jobs. Good healthcare demands the best of the best service, and care that is compromised simply means there are fewer people to work all the positions. These include not just physicians who have left their jobs and changed directions but also nurses and multidisciplinary support, who are the backbone of the system. Without effective incentives to stay in one place, I don't see any of this changing. Local hospital systems, such as mine, have tried to compete and offer premium compensation, but this has not yet resulted in stemming the flood of talented people leaving.

Being short-staffed has become the norm; I hear it every day, from many departments. It's a vicious cycle wherein we are asking our workers to do more and more with less and less, under extraordinary circumstances. Recent outbreaks and stressors are not limited to COVID: in addition to pandemic-related health complications, other infectious person-to-person diseases such as monkeypox and even polio are demanding attention. The pressure on our frontline staff is severe, to say nothing of the ongoing needs of our patients who are already hospitalized with complex illnesses. Many of our best and most highly trained workers are saddled with doing mundane tasks that can't be staffed by others. Burnout is increasing. For these and similar reasons, the future of healthcare is at serious risk.

* * *

As winter 2020 approached, dire warnings were issued at the local and national level about the impending COVID surge—and we still were without a vaccine. Though we were told that a vaccine was in the works, we were left with the same mitigation strategies as when the disease first broke out. The public began to feel exhausted, and pandemic fatigue had set in. Travel was picking up, and the holidays were approaching. People wanted to be reunited with their families.

My family was longing to get back to normalcy. Kaveh, now seven and some months old, didn't leave the house. He was not exposed to anyone outside of his immediate family and grandparents. Kaiya was good about masking, keeping exposures outside our home to a minimum. Yet, our day-in, day-out family routine had become Groundhog Day, ever repeating in a nonstop cycle. We tried to vary it with different hobbies and activities such as new crafts projects and gardening. Yogita was adjusting to the demands of her new job, which involved new expectations and a roster of new patients with different clinical needs. We were trying to adapt to our new family of four, with two working full-time physician parents in the midst of an outbreak that was coming in waves. Some days we were winning, other days we were losing, with cranky children and crankier parents who more and more felt as if nothing was going right.

For us, it wasn't so much pandemic fatigue as pandemic frustration. My daughter's fifth birthday party, for instance, had to be celebrated virtually; insignificant, perhaps, in view of what was happening in the world, but a little girl's milestone was tinged with regret. On another day that fall, we thought it would be OK to go to Trader Joe's—a rare outing—to shop as a family. We three could mask, but Kaveh was still too young. Naively, we assumed that masking requirements would be adhered to, since these were prominently posted at the entrance to all the stores, Trader Joe's included, yet that simply wasn't the case. As soon as we entered, we were stunned to see a crowd of busy shoppers with masks down on their chins and their noses wholly exposed, sneezing, coughing, chatting away, their mask clearly a prop to satisfy the requirement. To make things worse, this was the first time Kaveh had ever seen a grocery store and this many people at once. He instantly burst into a shrieking fit, screaming and wailing the minute we walked in. People stared, we were shocked, and on top of it all, we felt judged—by the very ones who posed the greatest, most immediate threat to our son. The family outing was a total disaster. We were out of there in minutes and headed straight back home.

* * *

On a Wednesday afternoon in mid–November, I had both children at home and a workday packed with virtual meetings, my attention being pulled in all directions. Kaiya was busy with her minischool while Kaveh was now active, crawling and exploring wherever he could. Every minute was full. Though I barely had time to eat, I got through it, keeping an eye on the kids and making sure they had what they needed. By the end of the day, I was exhausted.

Thanksgiving was fast approaching, and for days there had been talk about holiday travel. The plan was to have my brother and his family come to Atlanta. After all, my niece and nephew were responsibly masking and doing school in a hybrid format, and, most important, they all were hypervigilant and safe from a COVID standpoint. Our plan was simple: to stay home, eat, enjoy company and just relax.

Yet something did not feel right on that Wednesday afternoon, a week before Thanksgiving. There was another, internal voice perpetually yelling, *What are you thinking? No way can Thanksgiving safely happen this year ... you need to cancel—it's too risky!* Over and over.

When Yogita got home that afternoon, I shared my misgivings, what my insides were telling me against my own wishes. It felt like a battle.

"This is too much," I began. "We both want the same thing and are trying to keep it together, but cases are going to skyrocket, and we've come too far to get COVID. I don't think Thanksgiving can happen...." My voice was shaky and tears started welling from all the stress of that day piling up, trying to keep everyone happy and our holiday plans intact, while a voice kept saying over and over *It's too risky, you know it's too risky....*

No vaccine in addition to notoriously incautious travelers meant that airports and restaurants and bars and abodes were going to be super-spreaders. We couldn't do that to our respective families.

Yogita agreed. It was uncomfortable, but I called my parents and brother and explained why we needed to cancel Thanksgiving. It felt oddly delusional, this thought that we somehow would be safe and get through it because we all really wanted to see each other. Though our hearts were in the right place, our brains were still in denial. Thankfully, reality kicked in: we had to prioritize safety.

I felt guilty and angry. Was it my fault? Was I going too far, despite all that I had seen, by imposing such restrictions on those around me, who might not feel the same way? Where else had I been too strict? Though I consulted with Yogita, these still felt like unilateral decisions. Were they correct? On the other side of all this, I couldn't—and refused—to put out of my mind the degree of desperation and suffering that I'd witnessed of those struck by the virus, what it did to them and was doing to their families. I couldn't bear the thought of going through that with my own. I couldn't let them be the next ones to suffer. What if little Kaveh contracted COVID after this one-time family get-together? I couldn't live with that guilt. Also, I needed to model proper mitigation protocol in all areas of my life. Trust was fast eroding in the public sphere and I couldn't do anything other than to follow my own advice. As for Thanksgiving, it was disappointing, but canceling was the right thing to do.

* * *

As more and more of the population is exposed, a coronavirus such as COVID-19 will mutate to find better ways to attach itself to a host. It alters its structure to improve its ability to infect ever greater numbers. Sometimes there's a lull, those months and stretches when cases are low, and we begin to feel safer and we let down our guard. Then comes another surge, and it can feel as though we're back to square one. It's an ongoing roller coaster. Learning to live in this reality is never easy, and denial is a natural response. I never would have envisioned living this way—to break down and analyze my every step—but in the fall and winter of 2020, this had become daily life.

Chapter Eight

Vaccine

As the holidays approached, we felt a ray of hope with news of a forthcoming COVID vaccine. The FDA was reviewing all data, and as word spread through the medical community, we began to reassure ourselves that this would be the last major surge: the rollout of vaccines would bring a dramatic decrease in cases. That was our dream and our hope.

Along with this news came rumors about who would get the vaccine first and who would be eligible among our staff and workers. Some worried about the initial supply while others warned of severe reactions, suggesting that we make plans around the likelihood of getting sick. One group of nurses outright objected, telling me, "No, Dr. Desai, we aren't taking that yet, they can't make me. It's too new." I listened, of course, and though I tried to reassure them, the best I could offer was to lead by example. I would certainly take the vaccine myself.

Then something happened that I didn't see coming, simply because it had never crossed my mind. An African American nurse approached me and said, "Dr. Desai, how do I know that they aren't going to inject you with something different than what they put into me? This is all experimental. I don't trust it. Not me. They can't make me take it. I will quit before I take a vaccine." There it was: that lack of trust. Whatever institutional bonds I believed in and attempted to reinforce among my staff were at a weaker point than I'd ever seen or experienced in my years as a doctor. Trust was lacking even *before* the vaccine was approved. If this were true among our own healthcare workers, how many others in the general population would resist and refuse the new COVID vaccine out of fear? Mere weeks away from potentially ending the COVID surges, and already the prospect was looking bleak. This was going to be tough.

* * *

Masked, wearing a black headcap, clear eye shield, light blue scrubs and a white coat, I scurried from one nursing unit to the next during the third COVID surge in December 2020, my daily patient list full at eighteen, all of whom had COVID-19. By midmorning I had seen only three of these patients, each involving multiple complex issues. Reviewing blood work, X-rays and CT scans and then developing and discussing a plan to help the patient decide a course of treatment takes a certain amount of time, as does complying with the PPE protocol for each separate room. Throughout, I would typically be interrupted with pages from nurses asking for clarification and follow-up questions regarding patients who, it was strongly implied, needed to be seen sooner rather than later.

That morning, my mind was beginning to wander, and focusing on one patient issue at a time was nearly impossible. I was used to multitasking under pressure at the hospital, but I was beginning to feel groggy from the fatigue and stress. I was preoccupied, too, with how to make room for the incoming surge of patients who were filling the halls and emergency room beyond capacity. Who among my patients could I safely discharge? This was becoming a struggle.

Between the two nursing units is a waiting area that had been converted for socially distanced staff breaks, since visitors no longer were allowed in the hospital. The break area TV is usually tuned to something neutral, such as HGTV with the latest home renovation, only this time it was tuned to CNN—and the chyron grabbed my attention: "BREAKING NEWS: FIRST DOSES OF PFIZER VACCINE BEING SHIPPED FROM MICHIGAN FACILITY." Halting mid-step, I watched the big white cargo trucks starting out from the Michigan Pfizer plant in a convoy on their way to deliver the first doses of the approved COVID-19 vaccine. We had yet to know the schedule, but preparations clearly were underway for doses to be ready in the upcoming week!

The collective weight of dread and exhaustion was buoyed at once by shared excitement and hope. My grogginess evaporated and I felt instantly energized, alive to the reality that this was no longer just a dream. As I was about to enter yet another room to treat a desperate COVID patient, I knew that vaccines were now, this minute, being distributed throughout the country. I made a point of telling each of my patients the news I'd just heard, and while the details were vague, I had every confidence that the new vaccine would be available very soon. Some patients were excited, others declared it too little too late, and, of course, there were those who were adamantly against the vaccine, warning me in strict, stern tones, "Don't you *even think* I trust anything the government is about to do!"

To those who lacked all trust in advance of any evidence that might run counter to what they already believed, I briefly counseled that I planned to get it as soon as possible and reminded them that they likely would not have been hospitalized had they access to a vaccine. Most would scoff or else mumble, "Well, I guess ..." at which point I would change the subject. Despite such remarks and willful turning away, I nevertheless convinced myself that we were approaching the end of the COVID pandemic. As I moved from one patient to the next, for the first time since this started, I allowed myself to be at least partially at ease, knowing this would be the final surge. I could survive—we could survive—the current stress, and the workload that threatened to daily crush us likely would never be this overwhelming again.

* * *

That third COVID surge was the toughest yet. Our hospital patient census was breaking all records: the emergency room tracking board showed a full range of ages and complaints, and the ISOLATION column was always jam-packed with the red COVID-19 label. Winters are typically harsh in the hospital, but with the current surge, layer upon layer of complications was being added to an already overburdened system. More and more, the COVID patients, with their complex presentations and pathology, were garnering more of our healthcare workers' attention at the expense of the non–COVID patients.

The stories were all so repetitive. "Doctor, we were doing well until we all got together for Thanksgiving. My nephew had been out at a party with his college friends, and he gave it to us." This patient history—of getting together with one or two people who had not been vigilant and ended up spreading COVID-19 to friends and loved ones—was by now a regular occurrence. Others would share that they were doing well with masking and distancing but simply let their guard down for one or two days. It all boiled down to the same thing: people who thought they were not really sick until they realized they were, on Day 4 to Day 6 of symptoms, at which point they would appear at the hospital in distress. We would see similar abnormal lab values, chest X-rays that had infiltrates looking like classic COVID pneumonia, high demands for oxygen, and, of course, a great deal of remorse.

By this point in the winter surge, we had become more efficient at treating COVID, and most of us had developed a system for triaging and treating it. The hospitalists were by now the experts in identifying the sickest among our COVID patients, prognosticating outcomes while determining the best treatment. There was a weird rhythm about it. Some days, when I would sit to document cases, all my COVID-19 patients would blur together and become inseparable in my mind, indistinguishable, as all were on similar treatments and plans. To avoid mixing them up, I would commit to memory one unique fact or quality about each patient, whether it be what part of town that person lives in, what she or he does for work, or some other aspect of the patient's life. I would make small additions to jog my memory when it was time to write my notes, and it helped.

We would collaborate with specialists as needed, but the true care burden remained on the primary frontline physicians and staff. The hospital was still strictly closed off to visitors, almost without exception. Families and others who could not be present at the bedside were worried and frustrated, angry that they couldn't physically be with their loved ones. Those who remained at home in quarantine often were dealing with their own symptoms of fatigue, cough and fevers. When the patient was ready to come home, a quarantined homebound family member frequently would ask, "How am I supposed to care for my wife when I'm still sick? I can't even cook for myself, let alone help her to the bathroom! You just can't send her home today." Regardless, the patients had to be discharged.

Nursing homes were full and experiencing outbreaks of their own. Long-term residents or those in need of living assistance were often stuck in the hospital until they had a negative test or more than two weeks into having contracted COVID (at the discretion, conveniently not evidenced-based, of the nursing home or assisted living facility). Our case managers and social workers were exhausted trying to mediate discharge plans that were safe, only to find that many of these patients would be stuck in the hospital for extra days, even though their treatment had wrapped up. Yet none of this could be avoided, as we were merely a part of that intense third surge and had no other option but to tough it out along with the rest of the community. As isolated as we often felt, we were not alone. Every city in every state in the country was going through this.

Those who were hospitalized were, for the most part, too weak to advocate for themselves. Illness tends to make a person shut down, not speak, and wish to be left alone. With COVID, those tendencies are magnified exponentially. The feeling, as described by most COVID-19 sufferers, is akin to being hit by a truck. Under normal conditions, a hospital patient can have family members at the bedside noticing subtle changes and behaviors that can be brought to someone's attention when such and such occurs: not asking for help with eating, for example, and consequently missing multiple meals, or withdrawing into near-total silence when the person is typically outgoing and chatty. COVID made such helpful alerts impossible. This was particularly sad in the case of geriatric patients in their eighties and nineties, many of whom did not survive hospitalization. Their bodies were too damaged from chronic diseases, and COVID was the tipping point for them. I saw several with dementia who contracted COVID at a nursing home or assisted living facility and never recovered. They suffered more than they would have from a natural death caused by their underlying illnesses.

For those who did not survive, I can only hope that we comforted them in their final moments and treated them with the dignity and respect they deserved; even so, I don't believe that was true in every case. Being gowned, masked, gloved and shielded did not feel like the human touch and compassion needed by these too often desperate patients. Screaming through a mask to a hard-of-hearing patient who clearly had not understood a word left me shaking my head and filled with uncertainty, hoping I could make up for the failure by calling that person's family or contact. Holding a patient's hands with gloves and communicating through PPE is distancing in the truest sense of that word; even more, it is a barrier. Patients felt they were being treated as lepers or worse—as though they were the contaminant itself, as something to be washed off and disposed of, quickly. Seeing only the eyes of a nurse, therapist or physician through a face shield in full PPE made them feel less than human, that they were something to be examined in a petri dish, to be tested and labeled and filed away with a designated case number, a statistic. For staying at the bedside of these patients, giving comfort, the nurses and nurse technicians deserve full credit; at a time when the families and loved ones couldn't be there, these providers did their best to take their place. The reality, though, was that none of us could remain in these isolated rooms for prolonged periods. We were still unvaccinated and the risk of spread was great, even though we were masked, shielded, gowned and gloved.

* * *

One morning in the midst of this surge, a patient who was slowly recovering from COVID coughed in my face while I was examining her. Feeling that warm gush of air through my mask, I nearly screamed as I jumped back. For the next two minutes, I couldn't focus on the patient or what we were talking about, my mind wild with thoughts about what I needed to do next. Convinced I had just been exposed, all I could think about was how to disinfect myself under the circumstances. I couldn't simply abandon the patient or tear off my mask or remove my clothing. I had to finish our discussion and, with her, develop a plan. By the end of those two minutes, my mind managed to convince itself that not only was I destined to be sick with COVID but that I would be separated from my family during all of the coming holidays, my heart already broken over missing my son's first Christmas due to work.

The patient didn't even notice that she'd coughed in my face, and if it weren't so frightening it could even be amusing; still, it wasn't her fault. (COVID coughs are instantaneous blasts, no way can a person control them—indeed, this is one big reason for distancing.) The minute we finished, I hastened out of the room, discarded the mask, scrubbed my face and immediately became angry. The nurses were staring, wondering if I had been vomited on or worse. I explained to them what happened, and they proceeded to give me pointers on how to avoid being coughed on the next time, having spent much more time at the bedside. Though I had worn a high-filter mask, it didn't matter, as far as fear was concerned: I remained neurotic and anxious, and I didn't even think about kissing my wife and kids for at least three days after that. If I wanted to get tested to ease my mind, back then the test procedure involved taking me away from work for a length of time that I couldn't afford. Home tests hadn't been invented yet. I monitored my symptoms, and, thankfully, I remained asymptomatic. I continued to mask around colleagues and in public, because exposure to the virus means risk of spread, even if the carrier doesn't feel sick; for this reason, we never truly felt safe, and those of us working directly with COVID always felt more vulnerable.

We were not just battling fatigue. With the increased number of COVID patients flooding into our hospital daily came an equal, intolerable degree of suffering. To witness such suffering mounting in waves, on such a scale—the very definition of a surge—is emotionally draining for everyone involved. These aren't just cases. These are individual people. While the object is always to provide what is needed at the moment a patient is seen and offered care, the person whose job is to help that patient is included in this struggle, in all its details. Suffering, in this context, casts a wide net: not just the wholesale disruption of lives, but the isolation, loneliness, and remorse that go with it. And the anger.

Suffering was seeing patients succumb acutely to COVID instead of the cancer they had been fighting for years. This included seeing families separated, prevented from touching, holding the hand of, or even being in the room of, loved ones at end of life. Up close, we were witnessing lives derailed: from unemployment, financial ruin, dropped insurance, isolation and despair, all incalculable losses. It was cumulative, relentless, and categorically different from the suffering I'd witnessed up to this point. It broke my heart.

Forever etched in memory is me standing with an iPad before a dying patient, holding it up for him to see his wife say farewell with a Hebrew prayer. He was on comfort care with a morphine drip, death imminent, gasping for air. How did I become the person holding a device so that a wife could say good-bye to her husband of forty years? She couldn't risk a bedside vigil due to a compromised immune system, her only recourse the virtual visit to say a prayer and to watch him die. It was depersonalizing, seeing the two interact. I felt my lips quiver, throat get tight, eyes tear; by that point, the dying husband was nonverbal, able only to squirm a bit and move his extremities as he heard his wife speak. There could be no privacy for them, and I, the masked and gowned doctor present with an iPad, held in front of the poor man's face in the last precious hours of his life.

I couldn't stand being in that room for long, as the emotions—theirs and mine—got the best of me. I may have rushed them, I'm not even sure; I knew I had to leave before I broke down. Without a means to prop it up or a way to make sure that it stayed connected, I had to take the iPad with me once I left the patient's room. The whole farewell was sad and awkward. In the days before COVID, this man and others like him would've been surrounded by loved ones as he took his final breaths, without a concern over time limits or intrusive interruptions from staff. He died alone later that afternoon.

* * *

In addition to the clinical demand, the logistics and operations of managing yet another surge were grueling. I wanted nothing more than a smooth operation for my group, and while we had already done this twice in one year, I had serious doubts that we could maintain efficiency. There were too many patients in the hospital now, COVID was devouring entire communities, staffing suffered, families complained, and I was barely holding it together.

One goal was to keep the COVID patients *cohorted*, meaning they could be placed in designated COVID units with one physician assigned to that unit to ensure minimal exposure to the rest of the team. Throughout the course of the pandemic, I'd planned and implemented upwards of twenty different census management strategies in an attempt to organize and cohort patients and patterns. These could change as often as twice per week, depending on the influx of hospitalized patients, which was extremely dynamic and hard to predict. On those days when the inevitable occurred and some COVID patients appeared on a non–COVID list, I'd get frazzled and feel like a failure. Whatever system I'd devise to better position us, some new complexity would be introduced that rendered that particular strategy useless. Another would be implemented and that too would have to be changed. The situation was fluid. It seemed important to me to keep the physicians who were treating our non–COVID patients away from the COVID units, if at all possible. Some of the doctors were pregnant, for example, or had compromised immune systems that put them at greater risk should they come in contact with the virus, even fully gowned. Why send them in to see a COVID patient? As we tried to make accommodations that were fair and appropriate, it didn't always work out that way.

Doctors are trained to not make mistakes. As a team leader, when I see that something isn't working, my responsibility is to see that it gets fixed. When that doesn't happen, every minute that goes by is an intolerable weight, up until the moment the problem is solved. I couldn't fix what was coming straight at us, not as leader, not as doctor. It weighed me down in ways that were both demoralizing and paralyzing. The problems seemed intractable, not just which colleague to assign to which cohort of patients but the bigger picture: supply chain disruptions that were now a regular feature, delays in testing, and our newest, the issue of remote COVID consult.

Some of our specialists wanted to avoid all in-person consultation with their COVID patients, allowing for remote visit only. Such was not our hospital's policy, and their requests were challenging to accommodate. One of my responsibilities as a leader is to discuss any issue a colleague may have and to work with that person and others to resolve it. In this case, a matter of the rules, my hands were tied, but I had to hear my colleagues out. They would talk, often in vivid terms, of why specifically they needed to do this and expect me to advocate for them, to try to change the administration's mind, especially in terms of increased compensation for ongoing pandemic work. Sympathetic, I could only offer them heartfelt words such as "I agree" or "You're right" or something equally ineffective. It bothered me greatly because it wasn't enough. The problem was real, but this wasn't a solution. Not one of my colleagues ever faulted me directly, but I held myself responsible for not bringing this to a better, more equitable resolution. This was a high expectation that I set for myself and could not let it go. I became my own worst enemy in this sense, pushing myself to a point beyond reason, trying to control the uncontrollable.

With rapid changes come rapid responses, and while we couldn't control the high volume of patients who needed to be seen and treated right away, we could certainly manage ourselves in the crisis, and that included dealing with the families' complaints, which never stopped. We recognize the need to keep families updated about the status of the patient in a timely way, but *timely* is subjective and a relative term when a loved one is admitted to a hospital. As could be expected, especially in the whirlwind of a COVID surge, the physicians on my team were being constantly scolded and yelled at by family members feverishly anxious and desperate for news, which they insisted they *weren't* getting in a timely manner. Here, I knew, I could be of help. I stood with my doctors, and we could be unified in our coordinated responses to these often confused and frightened people. To every angry charge of "the doctor didn't call me today" and "I didn't hear from the doctor until eight p.m. and it was rushed and the doctor was short with me," I would explain, in a calm and reasonable way, that we are currently in a crisis, that the pandemic is real, that we are accommodating a surge of very sick patients and to get back to every one of their families with an update and a plan every day at a scheduled time would be impossible—even if it's the right thing to do. I would add that when the family contact is made, these must be shorter phone calls—and importantly, that this is not the fault of the doctor or nurse but the reality we all now face. Most families were receptive to this careful explanation, but some were dismissive when they heard the word *COVID* and *pandemic*, at which point there was no getting through to them. They remained angry, and there was nothing more I could do. I know my team, and I know their hearts. The complaints were not a reflection on their work, but rather coming from these family members' fear and, in some cases, ill-founded resentment.

* * *

During this third COVID surge, in winter 2020, I had an epiphany that changed not only my career but my overall view on the healthcare system: that our worlds in hospitals and clinics will always and forever be disruptive and chaotic, and that it will be years before we recover from this pandemic, if such a thing is even possible. I accept that healthcare will never be perfect, but even more, that perfect delivery of services in our current healthcare system is unworkable as a goal and unrealistic. True, we must do our best day to day to ensure patients are kept safe with a high quality of care, yet the competing pressures from pandemics and related surges, metrics (measures, that is, of quantitative assessment), governmental guidelines, insurance companies and other factors will always distract us from our primary focus: the well-being of the patient. How, then, to ensure that best care is provided? In leading a team, the ability to toggle between competing concerns while delivering the utmost care to patients is key to long-term success. I hope to motivate and empower my team to do similarly—that is, not to simply accept what is but to strive to create possibilities. While this continues to be a process, I am better more days than not. Thus far, it's the strongest lesson COVID-19 has taught me.

* * *

As the vaccines were getting shipped out of the Pfizer facility on that December Sunday morning, rumors were swirling about who in the country would be first to receive it. That same day, my employer assured us that as soon as the vaccine was in hand—and it required a complicated preparation—the hospital would be ready within twenty-four hours to inject those who had priority, such as the front-line workers, which included my team. Not everyone was able to receive it at first, and in hindsight, not everyone even wanted it then, but I certainly did and was eager to get it. It was the first weapon we had against COVID-19, and I was racing for it without a single moment's doubt.

The following morning, the first shot went in the arm of a nurse in New York. When I saw that image, relief flooded through me. At last, help was coming. I spent the next several hours incessantly checking email and texting my colleagues in administration whether they'd heard anything yet about when we were to receive the vaccine. Every state was on a different schedule. Georgia wasn't top of the list, and when we did receive our supply of vaccine, the distribution was slower. By midweek, we had yet to receive the state's allotment. I was beginning to feel completely left out, though it had been only forty-eight hours.

My brother, a dermatologist in Texas, was able to get his COVID vaccine that Wednesday. He wasn't even in the first round of doctors who qualified in their system. Why was Georgia so slow, and by what rationale does a person who's not treating COVID every day on the front line get the shot before me? I was happy for him but at the same time frustrated that the vaccine rollout had no national coordinating center. From the look of it, this was being left up to the states, each of which was handling it very differently. I was getting desperate. I felt I was losing out, unable to join the thousands of others throughout the country who were already vaccinated. My social media feeds lit up with pictures of arms being injected with the COVID vaccine and still I had nothing. I was more than ready to show my vaccinated arm, to educate and empower others to do the same.

Three days passed, and still no vaccine. This was an eternity.

Word was that we who qualified would receive an email that night, Wednesday evening, to schedule our shot.

By 10:30 p.m.—and no email—Yogita said to me, "You look possessed, constantly looking at your phone and refreshing your screen. Just accept it, you're not getting the shot tomorrow."

"No!" I snapped back. "I've earned this shot, and I'm going to be one of the first. I will not sleep tonight unless I can sign up. Let me be and do it my way."

I was obsessed. The vaccine gave me hope at a time when all I saw before me were losses, and here at hand was a way at last to check the devastation. Five minutes later, the magical email arrived. Through a series of clicks, I registered for my COVID shot the following Thursday. Going through the screens felt like securing a place in line for the hottest concert ticket on Earth. Within minutes, there it was: the very first time slot in the system!

The following evening, I rushed to the vaccination site, which turned out to be an empty department store organized into a smoothly run, efficient operation, one of the most impressive I had ever seen. Pulling in the parking lot, I was among the first to arrive. It was fitting, entering a mall in December, as though we were part of the holiday crush, with its typically long waits, beefed-up security and a throng of eager, bright-eyed customers lined up for the hottest must-have item, which for us, today, was the COVID vaccine. We were giddy with excitement, registered and waiting, chatting and fidgeting with our devices.

My number came up and I hurried over to the injection station. For the nurse, this was her first COVID shot to administer. I didn't care—I just wanted it in me! She seemed nervous and was guided by a fellow nurse. I felt butterflies, but they were flutters of anticipation. The official rule was no camera or video, but I made an exception, as this was history and I was determined to document it. With video rolling and selfies on, the shot went into my left arm as I smiled. It was smooth, barely felt, and after a fifteen-minute wait to make sure I had no adverse reaction, I could leave. That was it! Driving home, I was happy and relieved, thinking the worst of COVID was over. I was grateful, too, to my healthcare system for conducting such an organized operation.

Aside from a sore arm and slight fever, I felt no significant side effects after that first shot. A few weeks later, with the second dose, I experienced shaking rigors, fevers and body aches. I remember trembling so uncontrollably that Yogita had to grab an extra blanket and a comforter to help keep me warm in bed in the middle of the night. I got through it unscathed, but the reactogenicity was real for twenty-four hours (which was good for my immune system).

The first doses of the vaccine went into thousands of arms mid–December 2020, and the limited data showed significant protection after just one dose. It was naturally assumed, then, that vaccinated people could safely gather around the holidays. Among those eligible, there was considerable pressure to be included in that first round. It wasn't easy in those early weeks to find a dose available in the local community. Yogita worked in a private practice, so she was on her own to secure her shot. With help, following productive leads from online groups and community connections, she was able to register at a health department forty-five miles away, in a different county. Not even knowing if it were technically allowed, she nevertheless showed up and received her first dose on the following Saturday afternoon. In those early days of the COVID vaccine, it was everyone for themselves if they weren't eligible through an employer. She, too, responded well to the first shot and had a similar reaction to her second dose.

Hope had returned to our house. Still, acknowledging our immunocompromised parents and the fact that our children weren't eligible for the vaccine, Yogita and I refused to let our guards down. We continued to mask whenever we left the house and limited all our social interactions. As soon as our parents received their shots, we expanded our get-togethers to include the vaccinated only. As we waited for our children to get their vaccinations—that is, for more than a year—we remained hypervigilant. While the protocols didn't change much, if at all, in that time, it certainly gave us a measure of comfort to know we were protected even if we *were* to get COVID.

To reflect on what all of our workers did for ten months without a vaccine—and with nothing more than masks and gowns as they treated each and every COVID patient—was not just surreal; the fact of it was historic. To mark that before and after time, the moment when at last we were able to get vaccinated, my colleagues and I assembled a collage made up of selfies of everyone's first shot. This will be framed and take pride of place on the "vaccination wall during the COVID-19 pandemic" in our hospital. I often wonder if a hundred years from now, will people look back on 2020 as we do the 1918 flu epidemic, which, in that time, more than a hundred years past, also devastated an entire world?

CHAPTER NINE

A New Normal

With the end of winter 2021, COVID numbers significantly began to decrease. In the months following, our daily number of cases went down to the twenties and into the teens. Having been through three surges, we knew by then that metro Atlanta and Georgia had peaked and now were beginning to recede. At last, we at the hospital could take a step back and focus our attention on learning how to live not only with COVID but with a roster of altered expectations and novel challenges. Our healthcare system was never designed to be confronted or seriously questioned by the public in a health emergency. The pandemic and what followed in the course of three surges tested all the ways in which we performed our duties, including especially our response to shifting attitudes from a COVID-weary, increasingly hostile and divided public. The vaccine, which held out such promise, seemed only to make matters worse. We needed to regroup and address this development.

I continued to advocate for the vaccine to hospital staff and on social media—and most importantly, I would bring it up with every one of my patients. Even if they were admitted with a non–COVID-related illness, a skin infection, for example, or any other ailment, I would always discuss the vaccine. For some, I even helped book appointments online in their local public health departments: the websites often are complex to navigate and many of my patients have limited English proficiency. Others needed extra help in answering questions, such as whether or not they can get the vaccine if they are currently taking certain immunosuppressant medications. I didn't have all the answers, but it was empowering to be able to help them.

To be honest, I had never before so wholeheartedly endorsed a vaccine, even for the flu—and now, perhaps for the first time ever, I fully recognized the influence I could have in preventing the spread of disease. The responses were mixed, with about half assuring me they planned to get the vaccine "soon," which told me more than anything else they were watching for any side effects among those who were already vaccinated. The other half vacillated between outright refusal and staying stubbornly on the fence. I couldn't really relate to why one would want to delay vaccination, which was our only weapon, after the amount of suffering we had witnessed over the past year. In those early days, I held out the hope that we might effectively halt the spread of virus if a substantial portion of the population were vaccinated at once, and in any case, the sooner the better.

That possibility grew dimmer and dimmer owing to logistics involving storage and the number of vaccine doses in vials. For this reason, we could not then nor can we now, to this day, administer the COVID vaccine to our hospitalized patients. In other words, even if a patient decides and agrees to get vaccinated while in the hospital, itself a huge win by any measure, we cannot prescribe it. All of us scratch our heads at this, but it remains a conundrum without a solution.

Every year, however, each of us on the hospital staff automatically receives a prompt from the electronic medical record (EMR) system to prescribe the influenza and pneumococcal vaccine on patient encounters, especially if that information is not on record. We aren't there yet with the COVID vaccine but hope to have that in place as COVID becomes endemic. With every contagious and high-risk virus—the flu and COVID-19, for example—being able to vaccinate in the hospital is key. Timing, too, is important: once a vaccine becomes available, it should be dispersed in as wide a range as possible, and early on, before the outbreak occurs. Since the COVID vaccine was developed mid-pandemic, this wasn't possible, and in the intervening time, the original strain has had the opportunity to mutate. This is why we're still catching up in our efforts to mitigate spread (hence the "boosters"). For this reason, we need to be vigilant. COVID has not yet been eradicated. Observing closely and using every resource available is critical in caring for our patients. It takes a village.

When a patient leaves the hospital, appropriate follow-up may not be possible due to a lack of resources, as is often the case. While perhaps not on our official list of duties, understanding the social determinants of health are at the forefront of good patient care. Allowing for a patient's circumstances goes a long way toward helping that person, and many do need help. Access to food and medication is crucial, as well as the ability to make appointments and follow through. Health workers aren't necessarily trained in these areas, but the health of a growing portion of the population depends on our awareness of what is and isn't possible for them. The solution does not lie in just one thing; it's a total approach, an idea that only now seems to be gaining momentum.

For better or worse, the twin pandemics of COVID and racism in 2020 brought forward these challenges and inequalities in our healthcare system and will not soon be forgotten. While we may not get it right for every patient, I'm quickly learning that by using every available resource, every step toward treatment and prevention is one step closer to saving a life.

*   *   *

By spring 2021, not everyone among my colleagues and coworkers had received the vaccine, and we were still far from achieving our initial goal. Within our healthcare network, numerous sites were set up to accommodate all who wished to schedule their shots. My colleagues and I would be on hand at various locations to help monitor those receiving their first dose in case of any allergic reactions. We were also there to help answer questions. No one had a major reaction. The only effect I noted was a jittery feeling some people described within fifteen minutes of getting the shot, which dissipated soon after.

To talk to these newly vaccinated folks was highly rewarding, if only to be given the opportunity to express gratitude. In taking this step, they were doing their part to help end the spread of the virus, and with that, widespread suffering—which, to me, in a pandemic, is a shared responsibility. It was a joy to thank them. Within six months, the COVID vaccine became a requirement for workers in our healthcare system, a condition that was met with a mix of support, resistance and outright denial from those who balked at what they considered to be a "mandate": a word widely used to appeal to groups intent on defying so-called government overreach—and even, in some corners, a "deep state" conspiracy—to further divide an already riven public. For such workers, the solution was now a problem, with yet more attrition as a result. Despite these objections, the COVID vaccine helped to preserve our workforce. To me, it was the right thing to do.

*   *   *

On the home front, Yogita and I decided to send Kaiya to in-person pre–K for the second half of the school year, to get her ready for kindergarten. This decision wasn't easy. We knew she would be masked and we were satisfied with our county's mitigation strategies; we also had to face the fact that our daughter was not exactly thriving at home. Minischool abruptly ended when the teacher left for another opportunity. Kaiya needed to be around other kids, and we were struggling with how to manage two children at home for the months ahead. The vaccine was not yet available for children—certainly a factor in making our plans—but we were not alone in these types of decisions. Virtually every other parent in every part of the country faced a similar challenge.

That first day, dropping our daughter off at school, was unlike any other. We were not even able to go inside to meet the teacher and see Kaiya's classroom. Online orientation had to be enough. Pulling up early in the carpool lane, we were anxious and nervous. Our four-year-old was about to be left in a brand-new school where she knew no one, in the midst of a pandemic. Nevertheless, she marched fiercely out of the car and was met by a warm and welcoming teacher, who escorted Kaiya—masked, with backpack on, lunch in hand—to her first real classroom. Driving away, Yogita and I just looked at each other as if to say, "Oh my God, what did we just do?! We left our little girl at an unfamiliar school in the middle of the COVID pandemic!" We worried and second-guessed ourselves for days to come, but at least we were on the same page.

That afternoon, the first thing Kaiya told me when I went to pick her up was that her day was pure "amaze-balls"—her new word for *fantastic*. I was instantly relieved, but of course my very next question was, "How many other kids wore their mask today?" I couldn't help it. My persistent focus on COVID and safety protocols had made me perennially suspicious. I had questions not only about Kaiya's classmates but also about Kaiya's teachers: were they, too, masking? Fortunately, they were—and even sent us pictures of the kids in class. Most wore their masks correctly, covering the mouth and nose; some, of course, didn't. Every so often we would receive an email about one or two COVID cases that school year, a number that stayed low. Schools with efficiently run mitigation measures had moved mountains.

Kaiya wasn't the only one leaving the premises that year. A few months after Kaiya started pre–K, Kaveh turned one and became much more mobile and active. As COVID receded from that wintertime surge, it was time to start sending him to daycare—another decision not easily made. Yet to adjust our home and work activities to manage an extremely active fourteen-month-old toddler simply wasn't possible. Our little boy was growing up, and we had to show him the outside world, with or without a vaccine.

For Kaveh, daycare was less than amaze-balls. Rather, it was cause for his tears and angst every morning at the prospect of leaving us. I was haunted by guilt, debating about whether or not to keep him at home for just a few more months while we waited to see what happened with COVID. I knew that we couldn't. Trusted daycare was precisely what was needed.

* * *

Hospital life settled in to a new normal. Spring was here, the weather was warmer and COVID cases were down to single digits. The lobby now was filled with patients and their family members (thankfully, masked), a refreshing change from the days of lockdown and isolation, where every day felt surreal, like an episode of *The Twilight Zone*. At last, we had emerged from that creepy ghost town environment.

For administrative tasks, we were moving toward in-person (optional) and hybrid online meetings. For in-person, most remained masked (including me) but there were some who felt emboldened to forego that protection after having received their second shot. I was less comfortable with face-to-face exposure at the hospital, even among vaccinated colleagues; all of us took our own time in adjusting.

One unexpected benefit of COVID lockdown over time was the emergence of being able to work from home via online communication. This was new. Years ago, it would have been unheard of for a hospital director to attend meetings from home, but now we had to make room in our work for each of our families as well, since they were part of the new work environment. To do so required a different work-life balance, as the two were now merged, thanks to COVID. I was relieved to find that I had the support in both places during a time that demanded flexibility and skills to adapt to fast-moving, highly changeable conditions. Priorities included what was needed from us at home, and now that was accepted in our culture. My colleagues and I, working remotely, remained productive and engaged—even when such meetings took us deep into the night. Considering the alternatives, it has been the lesser of two evils.

At the hospital, patients and their families were still required to mask, and restrictions on visitors were in place. While the staff observed every protocol, many of our patients did not. Most had to be reminded to don their masks, and some were too weak and confused to ever manage it.

As the national spotlight shifted away from COVID—and with it, that sense of national emergency—our staff and workers began to feel deflated, as it became clear that shoring up the flaws in our system no longer was a top priority. Though the damages wrought by COVID continue to be felt, the media has moved on. Recovery is slow. We took a big hit. It will be years before we regain what was lost, indeed if that ever even happens. Still, we are expected to function at the topmost level, providing the highest quality care no matter how many disruptions to the system. And COVID, as we know, persists.

* * *

Life outside the hospital, too, was attempting to return to a pre–COVID normal. I heard mention on TV about Broadway shows reopening in New York, and that city beginning to buzz again; it brought up a host of feelings. I'd spent two years of my medical school training in New York, traveling among all five boroughs to different hospitals for clinical rotations. I'd become greatly attached to the city, as often happens during a pivotal time in one's life, and seeing it in lockdown hit me in ways I find hard to describe. Now, out of the winter thaw and with the third COVID surge in retreat, New York was coming back to life and filling me with hope. Having been first to fall, perhaps New York City, back on its feet, would lead the country to normalcy.

At home, Yogita and I were also trying to get back to some semblance of normal. That would include our going out on date nights, assuming the restaurants were well-enough ventilated and the tables not too close to one another. COVID had constricted us in so many ways, we were beginning to forget we were a couple. To be able to simply go out to dinner felt liberating.

As for travel, that taboo had been lifted, for now. We were eager to take Kaveh to visit family members in Texas and Maryland, whom we hadn't seen since the start of the pandemic. He couldn't mask yet, but by that summer 2021, while the FAA still required masking for travel, it wasn't a problem and we were able to do the trip. The prospect of reconnecting with family was exciting, and we could feel it surrounding us, this powerful shared joy. All of us were emerging, at last, from our cocoons.

* * *

As the vaccines became more and more available in April and May of 2021 and we began to move on as a country, eerie signals from around the world showed that COVID was far from over. Once again, we were seeing the ravages of COVID surging through communities far and wide, this time the numbers of dead and dying rising high in India. These were hellscapes, with horrific scenes of mass graves, severely diminished hospital capacity, and medications and supplies running out. The Delta variant had arrived in a wave, and this new predominant strain was in India. The country's border was briefly shut down, yet people continued to travel in and out every day. While most of my family resides in the United States, Yogita and I have cousins and distant relatives who live in India, and I would constantly text them for updates. They were in strict lockdown, I was told, and the cases there were bad. Vaccinations were sporadic, with some receiving only a single dose and many if not most without access to any vaccines at all. I would tell myself—mistakenly, as I now know—that the vaccine saved us in the United States, that what was happening in other places was due to poorly led vaccination efforts and a lack of access that allowed COVID to mutate. And importantly, since we are a resource-rich nation, that could not and would not happen here. Such is the power of false reasoning, especially when one is trying to reassure oneself.

The Delta variant appeared to be more aggressive and contagious, and in India it was unrelenting for weeks. Delta is a variant strain that altered the SARS-CoV-2 spike protein—the viral molecule responsible for recognizing and invading cells—making it at least 40 percent more transmissible than the 2020 (Alpha) coronavirus. That the original COVID-19 virus would mutate was expected, given how viruses behave; what we couldn't predict was in what precise manner it would change. The goal is ultimately to eliminate the virus with high vaccination rates so that the circulating virus doesn't have a chance to adapt itself or mutate into something even more infectious. Given that our vaccination rate remained low, this is exactly what was happening around the world—and also here, in the United States.

During this time, I continued to advocate vociferously for those in our community to get vaccinated—and soon. When the vaccine first arrived, I noticed that some held out, waiting to see what would happen to the others once they received their injections. Clearly, by now, they should have seen the effects, enough to know that the vaccine is safe. Yet, these fence-sitters, having grown in number, were conspicuously moving further and further away from ever getting vaccinated, claiming all sorts of reasons why they shouldn't. At times, it felt that misinformation was spreading even faster than the virus.

By late spring, vaccination rates had plateaued. In conversations with people, I would point to images on hospital TVs showing terrifying footage of what was going on with the Delta virus in India, but to them, it felt far away. Sadly, to many, this is simply what happens in third-world countries, and the United States will always be exceptional, so long as we preserve our resources and status. After all, over here, we had the vaccine. Isn't that enough to protect us?

* * *

Five months into a nationwide effort to distribute and administer the COVID vaccine, and still we had holdouts and those who refused to take it. On the cusp of preventing what was sure to be another surge, we were witnessing the rise of what would come to be known as the "anti-vax" movement, encouraged and enabled by social media influencers seeking to create a coalition of like-minded people through the exchange of both factual and nonfactual information. Poorly understood science and misinformation led quickly to widespread suspicion and distrust, in every quarter of the country. It had gotten to the point where, even among our staff, you didn't have to be a vaccine denier to harbor serious questions about vaccine effectiveness and safety. Mistrust was now a permanent staple in how we receive information. This is the power of media, exponentially augmented with every "like" and "share." We tend to listen to our friends and family more, perhaps, than we do the experts and public authorities. So, predictably, the campaigns that featured doctors and celebrities encouraging us all to get the vaccine were beginning to fall on deaf ears. How many, no one could be sure, but that number was substantial and growing. In the case of a new and opportunistic virus, that spelled trouble. And now, as we saw every day on TV, COVID had spawned an even more contagious variant. Delta, I knew, was threatening our shores.

Fighting fire with fire, I encouraged my patients to use their voices on social media, in their churches and throughout their communities to appeal to everyone to go get vaccinated. This, I would emphasize, is where good health starts.

"I'm sorry you're here with COVID, but know that you can get vaccinated after completion of your quarantine and when you're stronger again—which could be as soon as the fourteen-day mark," is how I typically would close out an encounter with a patient.

"I'm still not getting vaccinated, Doctor. I've had COVID and won't get it again," came the now familiar reply. "And, honestly, this wasn't even that bad. It's just like a bad flu."

I'd try hard not to roll my eyes and say, "Whatever! Do what you want." Rather, I would tell such a patient, "It's your choice, but our recommendation is still to get vaccinated to avoid potentially getting this again." Never mind that this recommendation was sure to be ignored—and that comparing COVID to the flu makes my blood boil—but the important thing is to attempt to educate, to break through the concrete wall. That myths endure is commonly known, yet what isn't so well regarded as fact is how many people can actually be reached. We need to try. At that point, in 2021, our vaccination rate remained lower, at both the local and national level.

Patients weren't the only ones kicking. Among colleagues, staff and other leaders, COVID fatigue had set in, even as cases were dwindling. Many physicians in my group would come to me and ask to keep them off a COVID floor for a month or two, to give them a break. We would commiserate about how it was getting harder and harder to feel compassion for those who chose not to get vaccinated. We were tired and becoming short-tempered. We didn't want to keep doing this ad infinitum. How were we to cope with those who were, to our eyes, deliberately putting themselves in harm's way? Answer: treat them, same as everyone else. Yet how was that fair to our other patients, who received less of our resources and attention due to COVID—and who suffered greatly as a result? It was cause of much bitterness. Hence those requests.

"Doctor, are y'all still seeing a lot of COVID patients?" asked a wife of a patient admitted with sepsis from a spine infection (non–COVID).

"I can't tell you specific numbers, but there are several and it isn't over," I replied.

"You know what, Doctor? I know it's not over, and all I have to say to all of these people who aren't vaccinating is to *not complain* and it's too bad for you, as you had your chance, and now you're draining resources and making it hard on everyone else."

She sounded stern. I just smiled back and said, "I'm glad you're saying that out loud because I can't." In fact, I was hoping to hear more of the same—in a similar tone—from our local and national political leaders and influencers. We needed more advocates.

Of course, we will always be there for our patients, but in the case of those who refused to be vaccinated, I never worked harder to garner compassion. Frustrating, too, was the low level of regard given to an institution and practice that exists to help save lives and provide care to those who wouldn't receive it otherwise, yet these very same people took it for granted that we would be there for them no matter what. And we would. Indeed, that is what we in healthcare expect of ourselves. Now, with the continued presence of COVID combined with a sea of vaccine hesitancy and fears, I would be lying if I said I did not lose compassion for those who refused to protect themselves and others, who then fell sick and arrived under my care. I was never downright rude and intolerant, but I wasn't always warm. When I knew that any talk of vaccination was in vain, I would simply ask the patient, "Is there anything else I can help with?" and finish up, with no attempt to persuade. The right thing to do is to try to talk through it, counsel the patient who offers resistance, reassure that we respect a person's choice and that, in any case, we will always be there. I just couldn't bring myself to go that extra mile on certain days. We were being stretched thin, and under those conditions, with the vaccine in hand, I wanted everyone to do their part.

* * *

In speaking with our hospital epidemiologist, I now understood that, without a doubt, if the vaccination rate did not improve for the general population, we were most definitely going to be hit by the new Delta wave. We should be prepared for another dramatic rise in cases and the near certainty of becoming a hotspot. I sought different takes and joined virtual lectures to better grasp what likely was coming and what we might do to stave it off or at least mitigate the worst of what might happen. Unlike India, here in the United States we had higher rates of vaccination and a better system for administering doses; my great hope was that we'd reach "herd immunity"—meaning enough of the population would be vaccinated in time to prevent a massive outbreak of disease. The reality is that more than 90 percent of people need to be vaccinated in order to reach that milestone. The odds of getting to that number before Delta arrived were slimming by the hour.

* * *

Summer had arrived, and we were traveling to Texas. The masking requirement was still in place for airports and many public places. The vaccination rate appeared to have stalled but the CDC and other voices continued to advocate for it. On the day of departure, I was still checking email and was stunned to see a message from our CEO to all staff: we had finally reached *zero* patients being treated for COVID in our hospital. This was a first since the pandemic started. Yes, the virus continued to spread, but not one single patient was admitted that day with COVID. My phone started lighting up with congratulatory texts and calls for celebration. I was certainly excited and felt good about the trip, but I wondered how long this feeling would last, and how many knew what was coming.

* * *

By the end of summer, the COVID vaccine was not yet available to children, and while most considered the risk not great, children did die from the virus. Yogita and I were anxious about it, and we continued to be passionate advocates for masking, especially in schools, where the issue had become controversial.

More and more, we felt we were in the minority, not simply about observing health protocols but about public health in general and what we needed to be doing. Vaccine hesitancy was on the rise, along with fatigue and denialism—at a time when an extraordinarily contagious variant of COVID-19 was about to strike. True, we agreed on sending our kids to school and daycare, respectively, but we still felt vulnerable, especially now that people had begun to normalize the virus, as cases continued to wax and wane. Long COVID, too, was making its presence felt—disturbingly, among the vaccinated as well, who reported chronic fatigue, nonstop headaches, cognitive difficulties and persistent neurological issues; myocarditis is also on the list.

One of the myths about COVID-19 is that children were somehow not at risk, that they didn't present with it and therefore wouldn't get sick. While true that when it first appeared, COVID largely manifested in the adult population, it was never the case that children would be spared; yet, in the public eye, the risk to them appeared to be small. As a result, there was no great public pressure to develop and approve a child vaccine.

For months, we'd been hearing that child vaccine testing and trials were well underway, but the dates and FDA hearings kept getting pushed back. Clearly, the science needed to be followed; all the same, it appeared as though priorities had shifted—or, rather, I felt a distinct lack of urgency for disease prevention for our pediatric population. I struggled with this, not only as a father of two small children but also as a physician trained in pediatrics. Most people, to my knowledge, haven't set foot inside a pediatric hospital ward, yet eyes open wide the moment one enters the dark world of serious pediatric illness. Ask any parent with a chronically ill child and I guarantee they will do everything possible to safeguard that child from the onset of disease. This is the point of vaccinations. The opposing argument, against vaccines in general but specifically as they relate to children, is that we just don't know their effectiveness in the long term against COVID and its constantly mutating forms.

My response is that we do know the science behind vaccines and their effectiveness on diverse populations over time, including their use among children ages five and up, and the majority have done very well. We also know that COVID has killed the healthiest among them, especially if the child coincidentally contracts the virus with another illness. We know too, indisputably, that COVID has and will continue to make many children seriously and critically ill at times, and for every child who doesn't necessarily wind up in the hospital, there's another who will come down with long COVID. In the matter of pursuing a COVID vaccine for all children ages five and up, I considered it vital.

In metro Atlanta, masking remained a divisive issue, with some parents protesting that wearing a mask impedes a child's social development. I noticed, too, how many among our conservative population refused to take stock in what was being reported about COVID-19. While I witnessed firsthand scores of adults in the minority community shying away from getting vaccinated, most of them had no problem with masking. Yet one only had to travel twenty-five miles north, south, east or west of metro Atlanta to find a different world, where masking was nonexistent and COVID seemed never to have been a thing. It was bizarre and disturbing. How could we live in two such wildly disparate universes, separated by only a handful of miles?

* * *

That November 2021, the pediatric vaccine was approved for ages five and up. Yogita and I watched our emails like hawks to make sure we could get Kaiya signed up right away. Of course, she was anxious about getting the shots but she also knew enough about COVID to want to avoid it. Excited, we were able to schedule an appointment with her pediatrician's office, and Kaiya was signed up to receive the vaccine on the second day it became available.

Walking in that office felt like pure celebration: balloons were everywhere, with a strand of gold letters spelling out V-A-C-C-I-N-E, and doctors with T-shirts that encouraged vaccination. All was so welcoming, the place was smoothly run, and the experience was over before we knew it. The shot was accompanied by a mere few tears, and then Kaiya was eager to pose for photos in front of the vaccine sign (for posting on social media, of course). I, too, wanted my daughter to be seen as being brave enough to get vaccinated.

The first dose was in, and aside from some soreness in her arm and fatigue, our daughter did well for the first twenty-four hours. The following evening, while wrestling with her brother, just before taking her bath, she complained, "Daddy, my chest hurts."

My heart sank. One day after having received the vaccine, Kaiya now had chest pain. My mind was churning with doomsday scenarios. In a matter of seconds, I was convinced she was having an adverse reaction—that something bad was happening to her body, and that she, our daughter, was that exceptional case of the child who suffers a serious side effect. I immediately catastrophized myocarditis or pericarditis (inflammation of the heart muscle or cavity around the heart), a supposedly rare side effect from the pediatric COVID vaccine. Every ten minutes I would ask Kaiya how her chest was, and she'd say, "Good." Why didn't I believe her? I incessantly checked her temperature and looked in on her many times that night to make sure she was breathing, my anxiety at an all-time high.

Yogita was concerned as well but more rational, as always. The following morning, Kaiya was set to play in the last soccer game of the season. It was colder now, but she was keen to participate. She reported no chest pain and looked perfectly well. I didn't want to interfere or stop her from playing, but I worried that running might unduly stress her heart—having already diagnosed her with cardiac inflammation. Yogita often becomes frustrated whenever my anxiety peaks like this—especially when projected onto our kids—so I kept it to myself for the first three quarters.

Now, at the top of the fourth quarter, while taking the field, Kaiya stops mid-run and clutches her chest. Panicking, thinking she was about to pass out, I jumped out of my seat and dashed onto the field, screaming "Kaiya, are you okay?!" All eyes were drawn to my little girl, I'm sure, my having created quite a spectacle.

"My chest feels tight when I breathe in," came the answer, to my profound relief. This was nothing more than a bronchospasm (tightening of the muscles that line the airways of the lungs) due to cold air and running—and she had a history of occasional wheezing. Signaling all was OK, I went back to my seat and play resumed without any further parental interruptions.

The game wrapped up, and Kaiya did fine the rest of the weekend. She had no cardiac complication, and whatever she was feeling was definitely *not* myocarditis or pericarditis. Curious, I researched the vaccine even more and could not find a single case of vaccine-related pericarditis or myocarditis in this population. I did, however, find COVID-induced myocarditis in the pediatric population, evidence that further refuted the claims that this age group was somehow immune from getting COVID. This not only validated our choice but left me feeling vindicated. Also, I learned something important: I now know what it means to be fearful of vaccines, especially when it comes to one's children. I know what fear can do, I know its power, its unflagging ability to unbalance reason—and keep one off-balance. In my mind, I had already diagnosed my daughter and blamed the vaccine at once. All that proves is that I'm overprotective, a loving father, and that I tend to become irrational whenever my kids are sick—like nearly every person I know. It also proves that the vaccines work. They are safe. For any parent, patient, or anyone still on the fence, it's never too late to get vaccinated. One child gone due to COVID is too much.

Chapter Ten

Delta

"Daddy, why does Kaveh feel warm?"

Running over, I could tell right away from the sunken eyes and unhappy little face that Kaveh was spiking a fever. Yogita was away that afternoon, and if not for Kaiya's astute observation, I may not have even noticed. I grabbed the thermometer and pressed it against his forehead. It beeped three times with a red flashing number: 100.9.

"Ugh!" I said out loud.

"Kaveh's sick, Daddy?"

"I think so, honey, but don't worry, we will figure it out." All I could think was that Kaveh had COVID and our whole house was about to go under quarantine—two days before kindergarten officially started. Kaiya was certain to miss the first two weeks. Sixteen months into the pandemic, and life was still as disrupted as ever.

* * *

That fall, in 2021, the Delta wave hit us hard. The fourth surge arrived before any of us could prepare for it. At the hospital, once more we saw COVID cases beginning to skyrocket, only days after that celebratory email went out, the one proclaiming zero cases, that gave us such hope. Instead of perhaps coming to the end, here we were with another COVID surge.

Of those COVID-positive being admitted to the hospital, most were unvaccinated. Occasionally, we would see double-vaccinated elderly COVID patients with comorbidities, such as congestive heart disease and other chronic illness that then became exacerbated by the new strain of virus. In such cases, Delta may well have been the tipping point for their heart failure or other medical emergency.

It felt like a broken record. Here we were—again—attempting to cohort patients, rationing dwindling supplies of PPE, trying to ensure that everyone observed the same clinical guidelines, and, most of all, having one another's backs and guarding against burnout. Rounding and caring for so many of these patients gave me déjà vu: their stories not only sounded familiar but they also started to blur, especially when these patients were asked about vaccination. Many would reply, often with embarrassment, "How could I be so dumb not to get the shots?" and "My wife is so pissed at me that I didn't get vaccinated; everyone else in my family did!" As much as I wanted to echo the man's wife with a resounding "YES! She should be pissed at you!" I'd tell him instead, in a reassuring tone, "Well, that was the past, and here you are. We are going to work together to get you on the right track, and you can still get yourself vaccinated." Though minimally rewarding, such experiences proved that we could help navigate most of these patients into healthful recovery.

Seeing younger unvaccinated patients admitted with COVID continues to be a good deal harder. These are the nineteen- to twenty-five-year-olds who arrive at the hospital with difficulty breathing and present the entire constellation of symptoms. This is the most maddening, as the progression of COVID to this degree is preventable in this age group. The good news is that we don't see a high mortality rate in the younger population, yet we do see the same persistent suffering.

"Doctor, I just started a new job, and now I have COVID—I'm not sure if I'll still have my job when I leave the hospital" is a typical story from my younger patients. Suffering in these cases entails not only medical but also socioeconomic repercussions. Even if they can expect to fully recover, many days go by while they linger in a hospital bed with illness that could have been prevented. Their lives need not have been derailed.

I wondered constantly if we in the South would be in this position had we better messaging and buy-in for the vaccine at the time it first was announced. This new Delta surge was particularly frustrating in light of our state's overall low vaccination rate from when the vaccine became available up to the present moment. The ominous implication is that the future of U.S. healthcare will consist of periodic surges of highly infectious viral outbreaks and that little will be done to prevent them from occurring or even to interrupt the cycle. I looked at countries such as Iceland, with a vaccination rate over 90 percent, which, at that time, was far greater than our estimated paltry 50 percent rate. To see countries and communities able to garner so much vaccination support is both fascinating and something to be admired. Societies that are frequently divided have a tendency to suffer more, especially at times when public health requires a coordinated response. Understanding is key. Here in the States, I sometimes fear, we are just too divided to prepare for what lies ahead.

* * *

The ongoing social divides became more prevalent that fall. We had gone through the combined pandemics of racism and COVID-19 in 2020, but clearly nothing had changed: our city, state and country remain divided. For me, these divisions are starkest in the field of public health, specifically when it comes to vaccination and masking. I also continued to see both inequity and inequality in access to care and services among disparate communities. Countless African Americans, for example, have been murdered across the country in particularly gruesome, unjust ways, and as a shared social issue, it continues to provoke controversy. Latinx patients who may or may not be legally residing in the United States are nevertheless shuttled from one detention center to another, caught up in a system with no clear guidelines. Whether it's COVID, climate change, unstable regimes or overseas wars, each has a profound impact in our respective healthcare arenas and continues to affect every one of us.

Patients remained on edge. I began to proactively give more time to non–English-speaking patients and those who live in underserved communities, if only because I could sense their insecurity and helplessness in ways great and small, whether they were not being heard, couldn't understand, or simply felt frightened and out of place. I wanted them to be reassured that they had a safe medical home with us. Often, I would catch myself using medicalese with these patients, saying things like "We are going to continue your diuretics, as your creatinine is okay"—only to be met with blank stares and falsely assuring nods. Seeing at once that I was not communicating, I would stop, sit, and begin again. "Okay," I'd tell them. "Let's review. So we are going to keep giving the medicine to help get some fluid off of you, and your kidneys are handling it great!" This manner of reassurance is usually met with better understanding and even gratitude. I made inroads with patients' family members, too, who are often shocked to hear from a doctor by phone, instantly assuming that something is wrong. "No, nothing is wrong. I'm just giving an update." Such efforts help to build trust.

Similarly, countless Latinx patients who are hospitalized, with or without COVID, need advocates on the inside as well. The reality is that so many in the underserved communities don't seek healthcare until the very end of their illness or when their health becomes too compromised to remain at home. For those uninsured, resources are scarcer than ever. In the past, before COVID put me more in touch with these communities, I would simply tell these patients to follow up with the local charity clinic after leaving the hospital, write them prescriptions and move on to the next patient, assuming there was little more I could offer. Now, though, I see how I can help them navigate such difficulties as access to information about their care, as well as counseling about diet and other health regimens, and also how their medications work. Engaging with the patients' families helps greatly with these efforts.

The pandemic has been a critical time for me; in many ways, my eyes have been opened. I see more clearly how black and white our worlds are, how the system still does not take care of everyone. To help remedy what for too many people remains a hopeless situation, we need to get back to basics and ask ourselves what more we can do to support *all* our patients. There's no magic solution, except to try harder, one patient at a time.

* * *

"God damnit! Don't fucking touch me, n****r!" yelled an elderly

Caucasian male admitted for an intestinal bleed. Yes, he was getting confused in the hospital and needed a sitter—that is, someone to supervise outside his room. The nurses had called earlier for medication to help calm him and get him to sleep. He refused to let them touch his arm where the IV was placed so they could administer the drug. I was called late in the evening to assess this patient during the Delta surge, when all of us were strapped for resources.

Approaching the room, I was annoyed and irritated that I was being pulled away from a busy night of caring for and admitting new patients to attend to a disrespectful patient on the floor. I immediately spot an African American nurse seated outside the room, clearly upset, unable to look me in the eye.

"Everything okay?" I asked.

She shook her head. I went in, knowing what was previously said to her by the patient. Despite her nod, she had the look of someone who just had the wind knocked out of her.

Moving to the patient, I asked what the problem was and how I could help.

Still fuming, he screamed something along the lines of "I'm so fucking sick of being here! Get me home!"

I calmly explained that he was too sick to go home and that his family lives far from here. I reiterated that he would not be discharged that evening. He grudgingly agreed to stay, but I would not leave until I called him out on his behavior. Though beginning to feel the effects of his medication, he wasn't too out of it to carry on a conversation.

I started by asking him, "Sir, have you been cursing at the staff and calling them inappropriate names?"

"I may have said some words, yeah. So what?" He answered as though he'd done nothing wrong, adding, "It's a free country, and I can say what I want."

I felt my blood boil. This wasn't the 1950s! I thought of our dedicated hospital staff—minorities all—having to listen to this man's derogatory slurs. In a firm tone and my sternest voice (honestly, it felt as though I were talking to a child), I told him, "If I find out you're continuing to curse and use inappropriate words to my staff, I will do everything in my power to make sure you're not a patient here ever again, and you will have to find your own doctors. You need to have respect for the people trying to help you."

Refusing to meet my eye, he said nothing.

"Do you understand me, sir? I'm letting my hospital administration and security know, and we will act if it happens again."

"Whatever," was his only reply.

"Okay, then, you will be monitored throughout the night," I said tersely and walked out.

I could see from her eyes that the nurse tech still seated outside this patient's room had been crying. I gently touched her shoulder and said, "I'm so sorry you have to hear this from him. I appreciate all you're doing. We will back you up—you and all our staff."

She thanked me and I promptly took the matter to the higher-ups in the hospital administration. We were given full support, and interventions then were held with the patient and the patient's family (all of whom were deeply embarrassed). The damage had been done, but it felt good to know that the hospital administrators have our backs in all such cases, especially now.

We need always make sure that our colleagues in healthcare feel included and equal in the workplace, on all fronts. I applaud the institutions that are dedicating their resources and energy to help build diversity and equity and to become more inclusive. A big part of my job is to protect and support my physician colleagues and staff with whom I work daily under highly stressful conditions; they are always there for me, and so I am for them. If ever there is disrespectful or discriminatory behavior toward these workers, who are there to do a difficult job, let's be clear that the patient is not always right.

While maintaining an attitude of tolerance and compassion for a patient who is suffering is a necessary part of what we do, there are limits to what we must put up with in certain cases. When it comes to any form of verbal or physical abuse toward our staff—which has become all too common, especially in the recent past—we now have a zero-tolerance policy. This is due in large part to the catastrophic events of 2020 and 2021 that weakened already fraying social bonds and exacerbated racism, giving intolerance an opportunity to flourish in a society literally gasping for breath. It took a pandemic to shake us awake, but too many still have their eyes closed.

* * *

"Don't worry, we will figure it out."

A parent's words—the best I could do, under the circumstances—to reassure a keenly observant child concerned about her baby brother. As noted earlier, Kaveh was fevering. I was hoping for an ear infection or even strep throat—something readily treatable, anything but COVID. Home testing kits were not yet available, and the only other option was to get him to urgent care as soon as possible to be evaluated. At that point, Yogita returned from her conference, and we rushed him to the nearest urgent care center. Kaveh was stable and playful but still spiking fevers, and now he had a runny nose. Predicting the worst, I'd already begun preparing for the shock of bad news, hoping against hope that the next words I'd hear would be the pediatrician saying, "Yup, that's an ear infection." Instead, what I heard from the doctor was, "Ears look good, and everything else looks okay too. We're in the middle of the Delta surge, and I've seen cases positive all day long. We should test him for COVID."

Yogita and I looked at each other nervously. "Okay," I replied, "let's do what we have to"—well knowing what a positive test result implied: exposure and more than likely transmission of COVID to all of us and to his immunocompromised grandparents. The nasal swab went in, Kaveh screamed, and we were told that they would call us in two hours with the results.

Driving home and awaiting the results was torture. My mind was racing with anxieties, helter-skelter. If the test result showed positive, it would destroy Kaiya's plans to start school that Monday. How were we going to find last-minute childcare? Even worse—and most importantly—what if Kaveh gets sicker, and also gives it to one of us, which means *all* of us, given the hyper-transmissibility of the virus? However diligently we tried to protect ourselves, strictly observing each and every protocol, we are still just as much at risk as everyone else ... *and if Yogita and I get sick together, and then Kaiya also gets it.*

Yogita knew what was happening and tried to distract me.

"What do you want for dinner?" she asked.

"A negative COVID test for Kaveh," came the reply.

She rolled her eyes and smiled. "Me too."

Her phone rang. It was the doctor from urgent care. I was having palpitations at that point, but then I see Yogita smile and breathe a deep sigh. She put down the phone. "He's negative!"

I was flooded with relief and gratitude. We dodged a bullet. My son would be okay. And we could get Kaiya to school. This possibility—all that had flashed before me in mere seconds, then played out over the course of a torturous drive—was a rude awakening, that we aren't done with COVID and that we needed both of our kids to be vaccinated as soon as possible. For that moment I was over it, that feeling of nonstop fear and helplessness, unable to protect my own family, yet the reality was that we were still months away from a child vaccine. All of us had to stay vigilant.

* * *

As was true in the previous surges, the Delta surge came, peaked, and cases receded. We never got to zero cases, and the number of our hospitalized COVID patients continued to hover in the teens and twenties—a sign that from here on in, we were going to have to live with COVID. My colleagues and I continued to talk with our patients about vaccination, treatments and more.

Around this time, in fall 2021, we began hearing from patients about a drug called ivermectin, widely used to treat or prevent parasites in animals, as a desirable treatment for COVID-19. This new Delta surge brought with it a surge of requests that was turning out to be a tsunami. It should be noted that, while ivermectin tablets are sometimes prescribed for humans at specific doses to treat certain parasitic worms, as well as topical (on the skin) uses for head lice and some skin conditions, ivermectin has never been approved by the Food and Drug Administration for the prevention or treatment of COVID-19 in humans. That people were demanding it should come as no surprise, but what did start to happen—shockingly so—is that some physicians around the area caved to the pressure and were prescribing this drug to their COVID patients. Some of these doctors even believed in it. Notably, too, several of our patients who wound up in the emergency room had been self-medicating with ivermectin intended for livestock. As of this writing, there is no available clinical data that shows ivermectin to be effective against COVID-19. Furthermore, ingesting products designed to be used in animals is dangerous. We discontinued the use of ivermectin for all purposes in the hospital and were left arguing with many patients who insisted that we prescribe it. As a result, our system had to issue official guidance that ivermectin is not an effective COVID treatment and that any physician who prescribed it as such would be certain to face repercussions.

So this fourth surge was not just about treating COVID but also dealing with the massive aftermath. In this instance, the aftermath consisted of an ever-growing group of patients who don't buy into vaccination, who instead believe in unconventional, often dangerous, treatments and who now were demanding that we offer them. Navigating these difficult conversations took the kind of time not easily understood by anyone outside of the frontline clinical team. Making the rounds and seeing fourteen hospitalized patients can appear on paper as a very budget-neutral number to a healthcare finance expert, yet what isn't apparent is the time, effort and mediation required in each of these encounters on all aspects of COVID treatment. I needed to make sure our system leaders were aware of these ongoing exchanges in the doctor-patient conferences and was keeping them abreast of what well could lead to an increase in physician fatigue. This certainly fit the bill. We hospitalists were the ones facing these crucial and controversial conversations with patients; they were always time-consuming and happening more and more. I was proud of my team, but once again, in the midst of yet another COVID surge, it was coming at the cost of likely burnout.

Too often, I would lose patience in such confrontations, and with that, all grace and compassion. I'm never offended if someone doesn't agree with my political views or my stance on certain controversial topics. But on this one, I didn't want to hear it anymore. "Doctor, why can't you prescribe me ivermectin?" was a question I no longer wished or had time to answer. Instead of the usual lengthy conversation involving deep explanations about why it doesn't work, I became rather short and firmer in responding.

"Because it simply doesn't work and is not recommended," was my new curt reply, at the same time biting my tongue not to say, *Because it's idiotic—it's a horse de-wormer and we are humans!* Others would demand monoclonal antibodies when they didn't qualify for such treatments, meaning they simply weren't sick enough. Still others, including those who were very sick, adamantly refused to ever get vaccinated, proclaiming, "It's just like a bad flu" and "I can deal with this," even as they huffed and puffed each breath from their hospital bed.

Compassion fatigue, like burnout, is real and had become an epidemic of its own among healthcare workers, including me. Clearly, the ongoing COVID surges and threats had brought out the worst in the best of us. With no way to win or please everyone, what more could we possibly do? Colleagues would come to me, desperately wanting to know, "What's going to happen next? Are we all changed forever?"

"I don't know," I would tell them. "But we will work together to get through the next surge and do the best we can." To this I would add that they are not wrong in losing patience, and if anything, I join in their frustration. Nothing goads me more than a leader who, no longer on the front line, naively and falsely reassures those who are, with bromides to "not worry and remember that we are there for the patient and to be compassionate." While thus validating and coaching my colleagues, I was, in fact, coaching myself, as indeed I shared every bit of their frustration and often felt disdain in similar situations.

Living surge to surge in a constant state of fear does not appear to be sustainable and yet we can't simply sidestep crisis mode. It can be daunting. As the hurricane passes and damage is done, recovery can never be fully up to par when the storms keep on hitting. One of the CEOs with whom I work offered a wise perspective. "I no longer make predictions ... it's going to take years to recover from this." This is the truth I now stand by. We need to assure our healthcare workers that not only do we value all they do but that the years of recovery will be filled with initiatives designed to sustain and protect them.

* * *

In-person school started that fall without any consensus on masking. I'd see protesters in surrounding districts up in arms against what they viewed as an infringement on students' rights and development. School boards were under a great deal of pressure, and within my county—and, I suspect, many others—parents were deeply divided on the issue.

In our particular vicinity, views were mixed, with most parents wishing to align themselves on the side of masking. Alas, a compromise was reached whereby masking was mandatory for a few weeks only (in the heat of the surge) and then optional. Kaiya was good about observing the protocol but was shamed more than once by classmates who asked pointedly, "Why are you still masking?" Anticipating just this scenario, Yogita and I attempted to coach her, but she was already prepared with her answer.

"I want to stay safe and keep everyone around me safe." We were proud.

Cases of COVID were being reported left and right in the schools, and teachers were out with it too. It continued to disrupt, but the schools remained open. In spite of all the controversy, I have yet to see a study or official guidance from a medical society stating that masking precludes, from a social standpoint, optimal childhood development. Too many, though, have convinced themselves that COVID is not a real threat anymore—which means, to them and others, there is no longer any reason to mask.

* * *

It was during that fall of 2021 that I started seeing a therapist on a regular basis. It's been helpful. Not all of my stressors or challenges are work-related. What I find most useful is having a neutral party with whom I am able to decompress, someone who may challenge certain assumptions on my part, not to argue but to reframe perspectives in a way that allows me to check and, hopefully, confirm that my analyses and personal decisions and thinking are fair and appropriate. It's comforting, too, to know that I'm not the only doctor he treats. I'm not alone.

I continue to think back on my mentor from residency who told me we all need therapy, at some point, in medicine. What's clear to me now is how many of us are suffering in silence. I openly share my story with colleagues who tell me similar tales of their experience, often leading to what they describe as burnout. While burnout certainly exists, I believe the issues may go deeper. I am the first to recommend counseling and therapy to colleagues and friends. It's a healthful start, a start to self-care, a practice with which I have now become familiar. There's nothing wrong with asking for help. A lifeline is precisely that. If it happened to me and helped me, then the same is available for everyone.

CHAPTER ELEVEN

COVID Positive

"Your mother had to come home early from work and is taking a nap. She's not feeling well."

These words from my father struck a nerve. That was on a Monday afternoon, following a busy, celebratory weekend during which both my parents had attended a big Indian wedding. It was December 2021, and we were starting to see COVID cases rise yet again. Would it be Delta or Omicron as the next dominant surge? I didn't know, but it didn't matter; either way, COVID was becoming ever more contagious, and here we were in another winter surge.

I learned from speaking with my mother that evening that she was experiencing congestion, cough and chills—all of which raised an alarm, considering how immunosuppressed she was from medications used to treat her rheumatoid arthritis. Yogita looked alarmed as well when I shared the news with her.

"Go," she told me urgently. "You need to test her!"

All my stubborn brain could think was that she's vaccinated and boosted, so it couldn't be COVID, but she'd just been to a large indoor wedding—and would be at great risk if she were to become sicker. My dad, too, was not feeling well and, according to my mother, starting to cough, but he wouldn't admit it to me.

I hastened over with two at-home rapid COVID-19 test kits that I had fortunately gotten hold of at a drugstore a few weeks earlier. The idea was to have them on hand should the need arise. Now was one of those times. Upon arrival at my parents' house, I retrieved from my trunk my secret stash of PPE hidden there since the first COVID surge, when such items were in precious short supply: gowns, gloves, eye masks—essentially a complete hazmat suit. I went in fully covered, as though entering a crime scene or the scene of some natural disaster. I sat my mom down, opened the kit, and probed her nose with the test swab. Following the directions step by step, just as in a chemistry lab, I thoroughly mixed the reagent with the sample, then carefully applied the drops as directed. Both of us watched the fluid travel up the test strip. First, we saw the pink control line, as expected. Right before our eyes, another line faintly appeared, then became so visible that it couldn't be ignored. There were two lines, no doubt about it. She was positive.

"Crap! Ugh! You're positive."

We repeated the same steps for my father, and he too tested positive. He was in severe denial, however, insisting that he couldn't be sick with COVID and making me prove to him that indeed there were two lines. My best guess was that they contracted the virus over the weekend, at the wedding, which met all the criteria of a superspreading event. In the minutes following, I began to flash on all the suffering COVID patients I'd seen and treated since the start of the pandemic. How severe would their symptoms get? How was I going to prevent my parents from being next in line, perhaps even needing to go on ventilators?

As my mind started racing with every dire possibility, I was simultaneously attempting to calm both my parents, reassure them, and get my father to accept the facts and to abide by the rules of quarantine. I let my brother in Texas know, and he was equally stressed and worried. They needed to be treated with monoclonal antibodies as soon as possible—which is difficult, due to strict criteria governing use, multiple steps required in obtaining them, and supply issues. (Monoclonal antibodies are man-made proteins that act like human antibodies in the immune system and thus may be targeted to help detect and destroy disease-causing agents such as bacteria and viruses. Monoclonal antibody therapy was found to be effective against COVID-19 and its subsequent strains.) My parents did qualify for this specific treatment, based on their age and history of being immunosuppressed. In such cases, the idea is to administer the antibodies soon enough after a positive test to avoid the massive cytokine storm (which leads to severe disease and even death) and give an intense boost to the immune system. Lucky for me, that night I was able to contact physician colleagues who could help. What felt like moving mountains (it took twelve hours) to clear the way for my parents to get this treatment ultimately came to fruition. They were able to drive themselves to a nearby hospital and successfully received the necessary infusions.

I was only able to do this after many phone calls, using every resource to get through red tape and filling out a lot of paperwork, even as a physician on behalf of two family members. It made me truly empathize with those who cannot advocate for themselves. What about those who don't have a clue about how to navigate the system? This is most of America.

Our healthcare system, as we now know, is poorly designed to adapt itself quickly to meet the challenges of a large-scale threat to public health, especially one as serious as COVID. When a group or agency constantly struggles in reactive mode, to effectively streamline procedures and make things easier for everyone involved becomes very nearly impossible. Is it the federal government's responsibility to make us all whole, to keep simplifying and organizing the processes? Is it up to the state? Whose job is it to ensure that the system doesn't fall apart? What, precisely, keeps it all together? Community physicians are struggling as well and often call us at the hospital requesting advice. What's needed and required is too often confusing. There are countless patients who most likely missed opportunities to receive needed therapies, such as treatments with monoclonal antibodies; other, more privileged patients get more than they need, often when they don't even qualify. (Disclaimer: I count myself among the privileged.) Simply put, those who lack resources are at greater risk. There isn't much equity in our current system. Experience has shown that in a series of pandemic surges, at a certain point, it's every man for himself.

I'm fortunate. Both of my parents did recover after their quarantine. It should be noted, however, that while my mother needed one ER visit for IV fluids (from COVID-related dehydration), she didn't get admitted.

✳   ✳   ✳

The minute we thought we were out of the woods, on came another surge. After Delta, at the beginning of 2022, Omicron appeared. It felt eerily akin to the previous winter surge, only now we had a vaccine as well as additional methods of treatment (which could be hard to keep up with, the list of inclusion and exclusion criteria growing by the week). Complicating matters was a season filled with flu and other respiratory viruses that were peaking.

Models had predicted that the surge, once arrived, would recede just as quickly, but this fact becomes irrelevant in the thick of it. These modeled predictions are guesses at best, and so many have proved unreliable. Frontline physicians and their teams, however, know precisely what to expect in a COVID surge. Perks, for example, for our frontline workers are critical if we wish to retain them; as noted earlier, the financial incentives to go elsewhere are great for trained nurses and those with expertise in related fields, and attrition is always a challenge at such times. Novel protocols that once were a burden are now *de rigueur*, surge or no surge: donning and doffing PPE, mediating lengthy conversations on the need for these protections, and talks about treatments (including vaccinations) that often involve a fierce negotiation. Add to this the constant risk of exposure to a hazardous and highly infectious agent. Being stretched thin is also now a staple, my colleagues and I facing unprecedented volumes and feeling the onset of burnout with each new surge. It can be demoralizing at precisely those times when group spirit needs to be strong, and frustrating, too, as there appears to be no end to these cycles.

The new normal has initiated a raft of societal changes, among them a change in tone. No longer is it considered recognition-worthy to respond to the demands of a COVID surge; rather, it is what healthcare workers are expected to do. It is assumed we are to put our lives on the line, as part of the job—if for no other reason than reality now demands it. What changed in me was a desire to find my voice, to better advocate, not only for my patients but to support and promote my team. If we deserved compensation pay for high-risk work, I would ask for it. If we needed additional staffing to make ends meet, I was empowered to implement it. Advocacy is a skill I managed to hone through necessity, as a response to internal pressures brought by the pandemic. I need to be an advocate in any case, but no longer am I fearful of retaliation or any ill will as a result of these requests. Effective advocacy requires confidence, resilience, and an empowered tone most especially within healthcare systems that may be ill-equipped to handle changes. To be clear, not every demand was met nor every petition granted, but each effort is vital and continues to be worth pursuing.

While the number of our COVID patients hospitalized during Omicron didn't exceed that of the previous surge, it nevertheless remained a burden to our staff. We stayed masked and vigilant, on guard against the virus. Home testing helped, but supplies waxed and waned, and two years into the pandemic, we still didn't have rapid PCR tests (polymerase chain reaction, to test genetic material from a specific virus) available to staff, if ever there was a question about exposure. More problematic, this remained the case even as several of our physicians and staff were out sick with COVID during this surge.

* * *

From the time of the initial outbreak of COVID, we have been facing many unknowns—not the least of which is, how long does this last? Do symptoms recur? Is COVID ever completely gone from our system? Time would tell. To date, it's been two years, and now we have partial answers. Having first contracted COVID and then initially recovered, meaning they no longer tested positive for the virus, some patients continued to feel unwell and were presenting with a range of COVID-related illnesses. Others, having experienced only mild symptoms, later became much worse. Still others never fully recovered and continue to report a variety of health issues, many of them complex.

It was neither simple nor clear. What in fact we were seeing was patients being admitted to the hospital for post–COVID conditions, also known as long COVID: a wide range of new, returning or ongoing health problems that people experience after being infected with the virus that causes COVID-19. It was the young, otherwise healthy patient that had Guillain-Barré Syndrome weeks after the COVID infection. It was others who presented with indeterminate neurologic symptoms and blood pressure changes, indicative of some type of central neurologic process, but in whose cases the work-up couldn't find anything diagnostic. We were also seeing many new patients with uncontrolled diabetes as well as those diabetics who'd had near normal A1Cs (or optimal diabetes control) for years and now came in with much higher A1Cs without a clue as to why. Upon delving into their medical histories and inquiring about COVID, we would hear these patients typically respond, "Oh, yeah, I had it, but only had mild symptoms." Yes, mild symptoms—followed by prolonged and chronic complications afterward.

I am still not convinced that we have seen all there is from long COVID. While I remain focused on inpatient hospital care, I am routinely in touch with outpatient physicians and specialists, all of whom report that they, too, are hearing a whole new level of complaints. Long COVID presents with depression, weakness, headaches, brain fog, blood pressure lability, cardiac ailments, uncontrolled diabetes and more. While not every patient sick with COVID winds up with long-term illness, we all remain susceptible. To assume that COVID is just like the flu, that we are over it, that we no longer need to protect ourselves and others, and that recovery is some sort of guarantee, from my perspective, is playing with fire. I've seen how much suffering can occur. The risk of exposure or the consequences of contracting the virus just isn't worth it to me. More than health is affected; for those who suffer from chronic ailments, employment and other issues become serious problems: financial stability, isolation and despair, to name a few.

* * *

"Hey, did you see the email from Kaveh's daycare?" Yogita asked me with concern.

"No, what happened?"

"There's a positive COVID case in Kaveh's class."

My heart began to sink. He was unvaccinated, and the FDA hadn't yet approved a COVID vaccine for children age five and under. We were so close in June 2022 and eager for Kaveh to receive it. We had done everything we could to prevent his exposure to COVID thus far. A two-year-old is simply incapable of masking all day at daycare, and from what we knew at that point, the risk was minimal. Yet, when we traveled, especially in and around airports, we'd insist that he wear a mask at all times. Similarly, he'd be masked when taken out shopping, at the stores, out for groceries, any place people gathered and traveled. When we ate out, we would choose to sit outside or at a booth or table with good ventilation.

"Okay, let's hope for the best," I replied, shaking my head. We both knew at that point to stop there. Yogita and I are both well aware of my tendency to become overwhelmingly anxious, especially when given a good enough reason. I needed to focus, to distract myself from worrying about this too much.

We went on with our weekend, and because it was hot, we decided to cool off at the local pool. It was a typical summer Sunday afternoon, with lots of screaming, laughing children playing in the sun. Late that evening, Kaveh felt a little warm to me. He had been out in the heat all day. While brushing his teeth, I noticed that his body felt lukewarm. Could this be a fever? In that instant, my anxiety was back. The COVID email popped into my head. *No, it can't be....*

Impulsively, I grabbed the thermometer, and moments later, read the result: 99.3. I alerted Yogita, who rightfully made the argument that he'd been outside for most of the afternoon, he was tired and also probably a little dehydrated. Other than a slight temperature, he appeared to be okay. We gave him water and put him to bed. As toddlers go, he is the kind who sleeps through the night unless something is wrong, such as having a fever. We assured each other that he would be fine and that one of us would check on him during the night.

By the time night arrived, I was already deep in a doom spiral. What if he has COVID? What happens if he gets really sick? How could we possibly quarantine for ten days, without all of us catching the virus? How would we get time off work? We can't ask my parents to care for and watch him, because then they, too, would get sick again—and this time, maybe they wouldn't be so lucky. Despite that he was sleeping soundly, as I could see from the baby monitor, I couldn't stop fixating on all this, and the scenarios were getting darker and worse. Sensing what was happening, I decided I needed to act, if for no other reason than to put an end to these fears. I snuck into Kaveh's room and felt him with my hand. He was cool, breathing calmly. He squirmed and moaned but was still asleep, so I scurried out as quietly as possible. All seemed well.

The next morning, waking Kaveh, he was warm. His temperature was 100.5°. Here we go! Yogita stared blankly and visibly paled. I looked at her and said, "It's time. We have to check, don't we?" I grabbed the at-home COVID test kit and prepared the swab, by now having become an expert. Yogita firmly held Kaveh in the rocking chair, and I got a good circular swab in both nostrils. In went the sample to mix with the reagent, then the drops onto the test strip as both of us stared. Almost instantly, as the reagent started traveling up the strip, two bright pink lines showed up. No delay, no fifteen minutes, his test was positive within seconds.

"Uh-oh," I blurted out, then looked at Yogita.

Her eyes went wide. "Oh no." Her voice quivered. "My poor baby."

COVID had officially hit our house.

* * *

We coached Kaiya, who was old enough to understand, not to kiss Kaveh or get too close, which was difficult and took effort on her part. One of the cruelest aspects of COVID in families is not being able to touch. Kaiya is emotional, she loves to give hugs, and she worried about her brother. We somehow were able to reassure her while reassuring ourselves. So far, he had low-grade fevers and congestion. With his history of asthma, we kept his inhalers handy. He was homebound for the next full week. Yogita and I came up with a plan (as far as such plans go) to try to reduce risk and to test ourselves daily, including Kaiya. Without much evidence to support the use of air purifiers as an effective safeguard against the spread of COVID, I nevertheless ordered one with maximal HEPA filters that Yogita picked up later that afternoon. Our plan was to mask around Kaveh and eat in shifts to minimize exposure. I ended up staying home with him most of the week, as my schedule was more flexible than Yogita's. Thankfully, I was able to work from home—and grateful, too, to have such understanding bosses. Still, I was glued to my computer.

I was diligent about masking around Kaveh at all times, even while I read to him and also during meals. He asked me, "You mask, Daddy?" recognizing the change. Fortunately, he made it through COVID without any acute decompensation aside from low-grade fevers and upper respiratory symptoms. We were watching over our son in quarantine just as we would a petri dish. I found, too, that trying to accommodate an utterly dependent two-year-old with COVID in such a space over time is disruptive.

Two weeks away from vaccine approval for children age five and under—and then he caught it. We were that close. It's true that my son made it safely through COVID, but we questioned whether he would've gotten it if he'd had the vaccine. What about long COVID? Was his asthma about to get worse? We soon found out that his entire daycare class suffered an outbreak and was subsequently shut down for a week during that summer, precisely when Kaveh got sick.

* * *

As the long week of quarantine was coming to a close, we continued in our house to test for COVID. We three had remained negative thus far and seemed to have dodged a bullet. We were vaccinated and were staying masked and vigilant at home.

On day seven of Kaveh's quarantine, I was feeling tired. I chalked it up to the stress of that week, between managing Kaveh and work obligations at home. That morning, my rapid COVID test was negative, so I felt reassured. I was exhausted and decided to lie down for a nap. Sometime during that forty-five-minute rest, something changed. My throat became scratchy—not the kind of scratchy that I typically get with a cold. It felt different, both sore and scratchy at once, and it was steadily getting worse. I also was starting to cough.

Yogita had taken Kaiya out somewhere and I was alone while Kaveh slept. Despite my negative test that morning, I couldn't resist but to test myself again. My body felt different; something didn't feel right. I got hold of two different home test brands. Each came with different instructions that I followed to the letter. I promptly swabbed and awaited results.

There was no immediate change in color to indicate positivity, but my temperature had gone up slightly and was now in the 99° range. Things felt as though they were happening in slow motion. I watched myself begin to panic, thinking, *It's actually happening two years later, I may have COVID.* Ten minutes pass, and I still see a negative test with no double lines. Five minutes later, things change. I start to see a second, now faint, pink line appearing on the test strip. I just stared at it, hoping it was a trick of my eyes. It wasn't. In a matter of hours, I'd gone from negative to positive, with two clear lines on both tests. I had COVID.

* * *

Here I was, two years in, maximally vaccinated, and positive. What did I do wrong? How do I get rid of this thing? I'm going to have to miss more work, and now we are likely going to spread it. I took a picture of both tests and texted them to Yogita. Her response was immediate: a line of screaming emojis in tears, distress and dread. Treatment was foremost on my mind that afternoon, and I was anxious to avoid long COVID. I contacted my primary care physician—who is also a friend—and we both agreed on a course of Paxlovid. I was warned about some of the side effects, but I knew of its effectiveness early on against the virus. There was an issue, too, concerning "rebound" with Paxlovid, but to me it was a risk worth taking; better to knock it out as soon as possible. The consolation prize at this point was that I no longer had to mask around Kaveh. He was recovering, and now I was sick. Like father, like son. True buddies!

When I got to the pharmacy, the pharmacist grinned. "These are going like hotcakes today." My doctor called in a prescription for Yogita as well, anticipating she would soon test positive.

"Why are you taking this?" Yogita questioned. "You're going to be fine."

She continued to test negative, and I told her, "When I get sick, I get sick, and it takes me longer to bounce back. This is my choice to take it." The goal was to test negative by day five, so I could resume work at the workplace and get back to my regular life. Two weeks of disruption were more than enough.

That evening, my energy level dwindled even more, and the cough became considerably worse. How could I have gone from feeling fine in the morning to feeling as if I'd been hit by a truck? It was awful. I'd taken the first dose of Paxlovid, consisting of three large pills. I was warned about a possible side effect, a burnt metallic taste, which I experienced soon after taking the drug: within forty-five minutes, I was tasting old copper pennies, a taste that I couldn't rinse out. I tried Listerine by the hour and drank plenty of water but the unpleasant sensation would not go away. That night, I slept poorly. I was restless and sweaty. My joints were swollen and painful. I had a 101° fever and along with the coughing, was now distressingly congested. Yogita slept in a separate room. I felt lonely and isolated.

The next morning, I felt even worse. Symptoms included fatigue, dread, headache, cough, sore throat, all of it. I took the second dose of Paxlovid. I was cranky and still taking care of Kaveh, as Yogita continued to maintain her distance. She was helpless and wanted to do more, but we didn't want to risk her getting COVID. That morning, we tested Kaveh again, who was positive on the antigen test. This meant that while he was over his illness, he was still contagious and needed to stay at home. He wouldn't be cleared to return to daycare until ten days after a positive test. That is the rule.

"What else can I do to help you?" Yogita offered as she prepped for work.

I said nothing. Instead, I just looked at her. I was angry and frustrated. Angry that I had COVID and frustrated that I was stuck at home, with no other choice but to keep on taking care of Kaveh, even as my symptoms were getting worse. I was physically debilitated with almost zero energy, my mood was off, and I desperately needed a break.

"There's nothing you can do!" I snapped. "What do you want me to say, that everything's okay, that I'm okay, go to work, I got this? No, I can't say any of that because this sucks and I feel like crap!"

She could plainly see how low I was and apologized, though really these were words of sympathy. I was just so discouraged; I also needed sleep.

My colleagues and bosses were hugely supportive, and they insisted that I stay home and take care of myself. While this came as a relief, I still felt that kick of guilt about missing work. It's odd, because I'm always supportive of colleagues with illnesses and family emergencies; now was my time, I guess.

That evening, after taking my second dose of Paxlovid, my respiratory symptoms all but disappeared. It happened eerily fast. The fatigue, though, and occasional low-grade fever persisted, and by low energy, I cannot emphasize enough how severe it was. I'm used to multitasking, running around, doing work at a very fast pace; my mind does very poorly in an idle state. Yet that whole week, I felt as though my arms and limbs were weighted with cement. Getting up from the sofa or out of a chair was difficult. Showering and making the bed would exhaust me. I succumbed to the fatigue and started taking naps, sometimes for hours, each day. Once, I even tried to force myself to stay awake, but I ended up falling asleep upright and woke with a painful crick in my neck. I simply had to accept that I had COVID and hope that these symptoms soon would subside.

Paxlovid, once finished, also helped to ease my anxiety about the possibility of ongoing post–COVID conditions. Studies coming out at that time showed that Paxlovid perhaps decreased the risk of long COVID. I can attest to how it helped me and would recommend it to others who remained uncertain or continued to have mixed feelings.

By day six, I tested negative, and my energy was slowly returning. I no longer felt weighted down, my dark mood lifted, and I was able to get back to my life. To my relief, after a course of treatment with Paxlovid, my rapid antigen test came back negative. Throughout this time, neither Kaiya nor Yogita tested positive for COVID, so at last we could resume a normal routine without masking at home or eating in shifts. Other parents were curious: Did we still plan to get Kaveh vaccinated, now that he'd had the infection? The answer was *yes*—without a doubt. I couldn't imagine going through this again.

Having gone through it once, I sometimes wonder what type of reaction I would've had if I had *not* gotten vaccinated. What might happen to someone like me, with vitiligo—an autoimmune condition—for instance? I know what COVID feels like now and how it takes you down; what I couldn't predict is what course this disease might have taken in my body otherwise. I stand by the vaccine. The unpredictability of this virus and the increased risk to those with compromised health is enough to convince me to do everything I can to stay healthy and observe every protocol. I can now only too well imagine what hell those hospitalized patients went through with COVID, especially before the vaccine.

* * *

Now, in 2023, it's clear that COVID is with us still. A range of vaccines are readily available, with boosters to help protect against variants. The tone, though, in how we regard the threat and rate of infection has changed. We've stopped being vigilant, the government has seemed to deprioritize it, and COVID is no longer headline news. The feeling is that we must learn to live with COVID but without any consensus about how that might be done. We have not yet been able to reach that point where people even agree on what's at stake. As of fall 2022, transmission has decreased, but patients are still testing positive, and tracking has shown a fair amount of asymptomatic spread. Long COVID remains an unsolved issue and people are daily dying, especially older adults.

No one in our community seems to be masking or distancing. My family and I have made adjustments, and all are fully vaccinated and boosted. Dropping off my son at daycare, I am the outlier wearing a mask. When I see the other parents and we say our hellos, I can read in their eyes the look that tells all: *Why is he still wearing a mask?* Recently, at the daycare's fall festival, Yogita and I were the only ones masked. Some people with whom we're friendly asked about our stance, and we told them straight out that we weren't yet ready to drop our protections, that COVID isn't finished, and that people are still getting deathly sick. Meanwhile, during all this talk about regimens, Kaveh took his shoe off, put it on the table and immediately started chewing it. One of the parents responded by saying, "Man, you're masking, but look at your son eating his shoe!"

What could I say? I yanked the shoe out of his mouth and just shrugged. There's no way to win everyone over. We make our choices.

Though active cases are diminishing, an urgency around long COVID has emerged. There has yet to be a focus in terms of allocating resources, but the medical community is seeing it. There are always competing priorities, and budgets are being squeezed. Some of my colleagues who were otherwise healthy have had such severe complications from a cardiac and neurologic standpoint after having had COVID that they are now on medical leave. I'm seeing patients admitted for such things as strokes or heart failure who acutely presented several weeks to months after a bout with COVID. While we don't have a specific blood test or marker to indicate that this is due to the coronavirus, it's truly one of those clinical conditions that is a working diagnosis.

Children, too, are getting long COVID. We long have known about mononucleosis leading to chronic fatigue; similarly, we are seeing children and adolescents with brain fog, attention deficit, and fatigue that can be directly tied to COVID. I'm not suggesting that we mask forever, but vaccinating and boosting is key. All must be aware that the risk is still there.

"Daddy, even when COVID is over, I'm still wearing my mask," declared Kaiya one day, recently, this fall. I didn't exactly know how to respond, because I don't want to mask forever, yet COVID isn't simply going away.

I pivoted by telling my daughter, "We will just see what the situation is and decide together."

The best way to stop long COVID from becoming worse is to decrease and eliminate COVID transmission altogether. The messaging therefore must emphasize the need for everyone to vaccinate and boost and to mask in large settings or whenever an outbreak occurs in a community, especially in a cluster.

We need to get together on this. COVID is here to stay.

Epilogue

Reflecting on the past three years, what stands out to me is the sheer amount of loss. The losses have occurred at every level, starting with innumerable human lives lost to COVID. From there it cascades, to long-term physical and mental health issues, financial distress, loss of infrastructure, economic and political instability, social divisiveness, persistent disruptions at the workplace and in schools, the unprecedented spread of disinformation, and, for so many, loss of trust in leadership. These compounding losses add stress to the fractures, imperiling our ability to recover.

Simply put, we were ill-prepared for such a pandemic. I state this not to blame any institution, agency or government leader but to bring attention to the factors that landed us here. As COVID is here to stay, a multifocal approach is needed. We know now what needs to be done, and that especially includes not repeating our mistakes. Inconsistent messaging from the CDC and other agencies, for instance, caused many to doubt their recommendations early on, at a critical time when people needed to align. We were getting what appeared to be conflicting guidelines, further impeding our ability to inform the public. In the meantime, people were making up their minds, and many decided that COVID wasn't a problem. For such people, there was no turning back. They weren't about to shift their position, even when their own family members got sick. Naturally, this led to a massive failure in mitigation efforts over time. We frontline workers were battling denial on top of COVID, and often, when these patients being admitted were questioned, it appeared that denial was winning. Whether or not a person believes it's a hoax is meaningless at that point—and still, in spite of all we do, what remains is a lack of trust. From the standpoint of medicine and public health, this is an incalculable loss. How do we get that back?

Part of the answer is to let people know, as has been reaffirmed throughout the pandemic, that without a solid and successful healthcare system, we no longer will have thriving and healthy communities in this country. Further, if the disruptions persist without repairing systemic flaws, we will be unable to deliver high quality care to those in their most vulnerable states. One day that will include all of us. In its current shape, the healthcare system is reeling from the aftermath of the first two years of COVID, made worse by pre-existing problems. We are perennially being asked to do more with less. This leads to widespread burnout among our teams and staff, with the predictable result that their lives become far less rewarding. Mental health issues among those in health-related fields are on the rise. So many have left the profession, and concerns are great that fewer will enter it over time. This is a problem that money can't solve. While fair compensation for high-risk work is certainly necessary, it fails to address worker exhaustion and shortages in every department. We can't be expected to continue to work with less in increasingly stressed and chaotic environments. More and more, we see shifts that stay open on schedules because workers are too exhausted to show up.

The stressors and competing priorities health workers face outside of direct patient care can further burden and challenge their mental health—to levels that may be intolerable. Such was the case with Dr. Breen and others like her, that led to their suicides. Factors that adversely affect a community directly impact healthcare as well. The steep rise in gun violence, for example, in communities now has spread to violence in the workplace. In the field of healthcare, this has reached a point where workers often don't feel safe. As the COVID pandemic wears on, we see more and more violence toward healthcare workers from our patients that involves not just verbal abuse but also punching and kicking—and, as we saw most chillingly in Tulsa, a mass shooting in a medical center. Among those murdered were three hospital staff. Many more were injured.

Coming to work should never feel dangerous or risky to one's life or well-being, especially in a setting where the mission is simply to care for others and help save lives.

The first step is to acknowledge the problems. Next is what our healthcare institutions plan to do about them. I wonder at the volume of needed fixes, and how best to implement these changes. To be short of staff in a pandemic surge is unconscionable. Likewise, to have outmoded systems of operations and failing infrastructure is a recipe for chaos. Wasteful use of resources, too, especially in the allocation of trained personnel, is an ongoing problem. Any changes will not be overnight, and the increased momentum to drive such changes comes with high risk: there are always competing priorities at the time that get in the way of planned solutions. To push too hard too fast may cause systems to break. And we're dealing with people, after all, who work tirelessly, and who are no less dedicated than they are exhausted; we dare not risk losing them.

The COVID-19 outbreak and its subsequent surges will not be the only pandemic in our lifetime, and the stressors and divisiveness felt in our communities will continue to have both a direct and indirect impact on healthcare and the workforce. We must think and plan now about the future of that workforce, of healthcare in general, and how we are to care for those who are so vulnerable. COVID-19 has essentially now transitioned to an endemic state, which does not simply mean it's like a yearly flu. There may be far greater consequences of its prevalence not only from an acute illness standpoint but the unknowns associated with the harsh manifestations of long COVID that will continue to be discovered in patients for months and years to come.

As a leader, I received my first true wake-up call when I saw how the current system failed to protect not just my team but all the physicians, nurses and staff. My focus must include the well-being of my colleagues, in every aspect of supporting them. We need to acknowledge issues at the time they occur, listen closely to our frontline staff, begin by creating solutions with small wins, and always to recognize our value. While we must align with the goals of the system in which we work, adapting and adjusting to whatever crisis hits, we must continue to support and invest in our workforce, on every front. On those days when it all seems too much and feels hopeless, we do it anyway. We are there for our communities and one another, come what may. We must, so that all can thrive.

Bibliography

Alfonso, F. (2020, May 30). "CNN Center in Atlanta damaged during protests." CNN. Retrieved December 14, 2022, from https://www.cnn.com/2020/05/29/us/cnn-center-vandalized-protest-atlanta-destroyed/index.html.

Beigel, J.H. (2020). "Remdesivir for the treatment of Covid-19." *New England Journal of Medicine, 383*(1), 1813–1826. https://doi.org/10.1056/NEJMoa2007764.

Bollinger, R., Ray, S., & Maragakis, L. (2022, April 8). "Covid variants: What you should know." Johns Hopkins Medicine. https://www.hopkinsmedicine.org/health/conditions-and-diseases/coronavirus/a-new-strain-of-coronavirus-what-you-should-know.

Center for Drug Evaluation and Research. (2020, July 1). "FDA cautions use of hydroxy-chloroquine/chloroquine for covid-19." U.S. Food and Drug Administration. https://www.fda.gov/drugs/drug-safety-and-availability/fda-cautions-against-use-hydroxychloroquine-or-chloroquine-covid-19-outside-hospital-setting-or.

FDA. (2021, December 10). "Why you should not use ivermectin to treat or prevent COVID-19." U.S. Food and Drug Administration. Retrieved December 14, 2022, https://www.fda.gov/consumers/consumer-updates/why-you-should-not-use-ivermectin-treat-or-prevent-covid-19.

Hill, L., & Artiga, S. (2022, August 22). "Covid-19 cases and deaths by Race/ethnicity: Current data and changes over time." KFF. https://www.kff.org/coronavirus-covid-19/issue-brief/covid-19-cases-and-deaths-by-race-ethnicity-current-data-and-changes-over-time/.

Holcombe, M., & Levenson, E. (2020, December 14). "Covid-19 vaccine en route to every state as health officials say they hope immunizations begin Monday." CNN. https://www.cnn.com/2020/12/13/health/us-coronavirus-sunday/index.html.

IDSA Home. (2022, August 4). "Anti-SARS-cov-2 monoclonal antibodies." Retrieved December 14, 2022, from https://www.idsociety.org/covid-19-real-time-learning-network/therapeutics-and-interventions/monoclonal-antibodies/.

Knoll, C., Watkins, A., & Rothfeld, M. (2020, July 11). "I couldn't do anything': The virus and an E.R. doctor's suicide." *New York Times.* https://www.nytimes.com/2020/07/11/nyregion/lorna-breen-suicide-coronavirus.html.

McWilliams, K. (2021, November 19). "The Day I Passed for White." *Time.* https://time.com/6116209/passing-for-white/.

Schumaker, E. (2020, September 22). "Timeline: How coronavirus got started." ABC News. https://abcnews.go.com/Health/timeline-coronavirus-started/story?id=69435165.

"What is coronavirus?" (2022, July 29). Johns Hopkins Medicine. Retrieved December 14, 2022, from https://www.hopkinsmedicine.org/health/conditions-and-diseases/coronavirus.

Index